Praise for *The Rested Child*

"A fantastic no-nonsense guide to how to recognize why your child is not sleeping well and, more importantly, how to fix it. Rooted firmly in the science of sleep, presented in a highly entertaining manner."

—Dr. Guy Leschziner, neurologist, sleep specialist, and author of
The Nocturnal Brain: Nightmares, Neuroscience, and the Secret World of Sleep

"*The Rested Child* is without doubt the best book ever written on children and sleep. Everything you MUST know about your child's sleep is under these covers. Dr. Chris Winter's pearls of wisdom are invaluable, based on the science of sleep medicine and his years of clinical experience. He provides detailed descriptions of all child sleep problems and offers concrete solutions and parental action plans for the more than 40 percent of our children who will experience a sleep disorder (and the 70 percent of college students who are sleep-deprived walking zombies). This insightful sleep doctor's instructions will inform and reassure every parent who has any concern about their child's sleep from in utero through graduate school and beyond. He tells us how good sleep can be accurately measured and how it will improve immunity, mood, cognitive functioning, academic performance, athleticism, safety, general well-being, and life span. Dr. Winter's writing style is extremely fluid, warm, and empathetic. His treatment instructions are clear and effective, and his sense of humor, while dealing with a serious topic, is hilarious and will keep you wide awake."

—Dr. James B. Maas, Stephen H. Weiss Presidential Fellow,
former professor and chair of psychology at Cornell University,
and coauthor of *Sleep for Success!* and *Sleep to Win!*

"I so enjoyed this book. I found myself laughing out loud and nodding, and for this pediatric sleep doc who's been the field for fifteen years, it was joyfully eye-opening!"

—Lewis J. Kass, MD, medical director,
Pediatric Sleep Disorders Center at Norwalk Hospital

T0187024

"With a unique approach, Dr. Christopher Winter manages to make the important topic of children and sleep engaging. A must-read for parents who want to understand and improve their children's sleep health and the important role they play. I highly recommend this book. I know I couldn't put it down!"

—Suzy Giordano, coauthor of *Twelve Hours' Sleep at Twelve Weeks Old* and *The Baby Sleep Solution*

"Sleep is as important to health as breathing and eating, and yet sleep problems are often mysterious to parents and pediatricians alike. In Chris Winter's insightful and funny new book, *The Rested Child*, he provides a terrific overview of the many ways sleep can go wrong for children, as well as a road map for how to help them. "

—Craig Canapari, MD, director, Yale Pediatric Sleep Center, and author of *It's Never Too Late to Sleep Train*

"Absorbing, immensely informative, and highly readable for concerned parents. Five stars for the bedside manner that Chris Winter brings to *The Rested Child*, a vitally important book for the well-being of our children."

—A. Roger Ekirch, author of *At Day's Close: Night in Times Past*

"As a journalist and mom of three, I have benefited both professionally and personally from the incredible knowledge of Dr. Winter. He has a unique way of making the science of sleep easy to understand and fun to learn! Plus he's a father who has treated high-caliber athletes (including "the American mother") so he has the practical experience to provide real solutions that can change your life. Dr. Winter helped me create healthy family sleep habits that have lasted for years—I'm overjoyed that so many more parents can share in his strategy *and* get a good night's sleep!"

—Jenna Lee, journalist and founder of SmartHER News

The Rested Child

The Rested Child

Why Your Tired, Wired,
or Irritable Child May Have a
Sleep Disorder—and How to Help

W. Chris Winter, MD

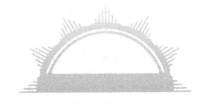

sheldon **PRESS**

Published in the United States by Avery,
an imprint of Penguin Random House LLC, New York.

First published in Great Britain by Sheldon Press in 2021
An imprint of John Murray Press
A division of Hodder & Stoughton Ltd,
An Hachette UK company

1

This book is for information or educational purposes only and is not intended to act as a
substitute for medical advice or treatment. Any person with a condition requiring medical
attention should consult a qualified medical practitioner or suitable therapist.

A CIP catalogue record for this title is available from the British Library

Paperback ISBN 9781529359695
eBook ISBN 9781529359718

Printed and bound in Great Britain by Clays Ltd, Elcograf S.p.A.

John Murray Press policy is to use papers that are natural, renewable and recyclable
products and made from wood grown in sustainable forests. The logging and
manufacturing processes are expected to conform to the environmental regulations of the
country of origin.

John Murray Press
Carmelite House
50 Victoria Embankment
London EC4Y 0DZ

www.sheldonpress.co.uk

This book is dedicated to the many kids I've had the privilege to treat over the years, and to Maeve, Tyce, and Cam—the three sleepyheads I had the fortune to wake up every morning.

Contents

Preface

As I write *The Rested Child*, COVID-19 continues to wage war on communities around the globe. It is a stressful time, particularly for kids. My clinic schedule is packed with patients with sleep issues, often fueled by their anxieties. This is particularly true for young people who thrive on social interaction, exercise, and routines. The lack of organized, predictable activities wreaks havoc on their sleep, which makes them even more anxious. In addition, they are also staying up late to play video games with their friends and to Zoom with the West Coast family. For my patients who suffer from excessive sleepiness, they are struggling in very different ways. The absence of a normally unrelenting schedule allows them the freedom to make their own rules and schedules, sleep more, and sleep more often. As life begins to move back to normal, these kids are finding it difficult to readjust to normal schedules. For most, sleep is complicated in "normal times," let alone during a global pandemic.

When I wrote my first book, *The Sleep Solution—Why Your Sleep Is Broken and How to Fix It*, I quickly realized that I did not have room to cover kids and their sleep problems. I wrestled with this. How can I put a book out there about sleep that does not address anyone not legally able to buy beer? I see children in my sleep clinic all the time. In fact, about 15 to 20 percent of my patients are children, including college-aged students who float between the youth and adult worlds. As I considered adding a chapter about children, I simply could not edit down all the things I wanted to talk about, so I began a new file called "KidSleep" and quickly filled it with the fascinating observations and researched complexities of sleep in children and teens.

I've always been drawn to helping kids. Leading up to medical school, I was fairly certain I would become a pediatrician. I worked as a camp counselor for kids with medical needs, volunteered with youth organizations, and acted like a child well into my adult years, so making the decision to help them out as an MD was easy. Over time, despite ultimately being pulled toward sleep and neurology, treating children became a substantial part of my practice and a coveted aspect of my job. I just had no idea how much of my time would end up unraveling the sleep issues of children, from babies and elementary-aged youths to teens and college-aged adolescents.

And no wonder. Sleep disorders in children are on the rise, and all too often these disorders are undiagnosed. It has been estimated that 10 percent of children have a diagnosable sleep disorder, but more than half of all children who display signs of a sleep issue are not diagnosed properly. Every year, children are treated for diseases like diabetes, learning disorders, and chronic pain, when the root cause of their ailment may actually be a sleep disorder for which they are not being treated. Even if a child happens to be lucky enough to receive a proper diagnosis, according to a 2014 study looking at sleep disorders in children, only 5 percent of those with a recognized sleep problem or disorder received any therapy for their condition. For children struggling with mental health issues, the percentage of those dealing with sleep disorders balloons up to as much as 75 percent. Often the sleep disorder is contributing to (or masquerading as) the psychiatric problem. That's right. Many families are waging a war with a disorder that is not the real enemy. It gets worse. Research shows that epidemic levels of childhood obesity, diabetes, learning and attention disorders, and more mysterious pain and fatigue maladies in children are deeply rooted in sleep. In other words, parents (and doctors) who are desperately trying to fix their child's sleep problems by treating his chronic pain with opioids may have the problem totally reversed—it's the sleep disorder causing the pain. The parade of mental, physical, social, and educational consequences of these disorders is almost beyond comprehension.

Sleep disorders are an urgent health matter that have received far too little attention. Moreover, we are in the midst of what has been called a modern plague of chronic sleep loss in our society, and children are not exempt. In 2018, experts at the National Health Service in England pronounced sleeplessness in children a "hidden health crisis." The number of children with sleep disorders, converging with factors inhibiting good quality sleep and intersecting with insufficient and inadequately trained providers, creates a perfect storm and is generating a sleep emergency in our children. We are losing battles against ADHD, diabetes, depression, and obesity, but all the while these diseases are quietly being caused by or fueled by unrecognized and untreated sleep disorders.

The perception is that these sleep conditions are rare. Nothing is further from the truth. The National Sleep Foundation estimates that two out of every three children in the United States will experience some type of sleep problem before they reach adulthood. Compared to the number of children who will have sleep problems (40 percent, conservatively), consider the numbers of disorders commonly thought of as being prevalent in kids:

- Diabetes affects 0.25 percent of children age nineteen or younger.

- ADHD affects 9.4 percent of children.

- Depression affects up to 4 to 5 percent of children.

- Obesity affects 18.5 percent of children ages six to eleven.

Consider also these statistics—the National Sleep Foundation recommends eight and a half to nine hours of sleep for teenagers, but fewer than 20 percent are meeting that goal, and 40 percent report high amounts of sleepiness as a result. A Fairfax, Virginia, study concluded that only 6 percent of tenth graders and 3 percent of twelfth graders are meeting the minimum sleep requirement goals. Given the statistic that teens are responsible for 50 percent of drowsy-driving automobile accidents in the United States, this issue alone makes sleep a true public health crisis.

Hopefully, I have your attention and I've adequately made my case for why I wanted to write this book. This is scary stuff. However, unlike a lot of what is going on in the world right now, the sleep piece of the puzzle is under our control and is usually an easy fix. My examination of sleep in *The Rested Child* focuses on how sleep looks normally throughout the developmental stages of a child's life, how it can go wrong, and how to right the ship. Despite the severity of the issue, I hope that I've written a book that is enjoyable to read, relatable, and, most of all, helpful.

Introduction

Before we begin the book, I think it would be fun to take a quick true/false quiz. Your teens take tests almost every day. It only seems fair. Good news! It won't be graded. Bad news! It's not open book. The answers are at the end of this introduction.

True/False Some children simply can't sleep.

True/False To get a child to sleep, a parent needs to let their child "cry it out."

True/False Kids in school need at least ten hours of sleep every night.

True/False Younger children always need more sleep than older children.

True/False If a teenager complains that it is taking him four hours to fall asleep, the perception is virtually always an accurate assessment.

True/False Growing pains, when present, are always a normal part of a child's maturation process.

True/False   Sleeping with a baby is a good way to ensure his safety.

True/False   Napping is essential for all children.

True/False   Falling asleep in class is an indication that a child is staying up too late and needs more sleep.

True/False   With rising technology interference, children today sleep less than children twenty-five years ago.

True/False   Ten percent of infants have some degree of sleep dysfunction.

True/False   Children who awaken frequently during the night or have poor-quality sleep benefit from more time in bed.

True/False   The effect of electronics/screen time on children and their sleep can be eliminated by dimming the light emitted from the screens and adjusting the light.

True/False   Limiting screen time is the best way to minimize the impact of electronics on sleep in kids.

True/False   Students who are "night owls" and prefer to stay up late have a lower incidence of sleep issues and typically feel less of a need to consume caffeine.

True/False   The health consequences of inadequate sleep in preschoolers can be made up for with more napping and longer weekend sleep periods.

True/False   Excessive daytime sleepiness is relatively rare in children and tends to become more common in adulthood.

It's time to talk about children and how they sleep. There is a lot of misinformation out there about the topic. One of my mentors during my sleep medicine fellowship proclaimed the highly unscientific, yet seemingly accurate statistic, "Ninety-nine percent of all kids' sleep problems are parent sleep problems." He said it all the time. That's probably a bit of an exaggeration, but he wasn't entirely wrong. Prepare yourself for some parental reflection. It's okay—we all think we know what we are doing as parents, but there are some things you simply aren't aware of. How can you know about a topic if you've never been educated about it?

From the textbook on pediatric sleep I was given as a gift when I graduated from my fellowship program to the many books written by individuals whose only pediatric sleep qualification seems to be a working knowledge of Microsoft Word, I've read a bunch of books that address kids and their sleep. While their messages, style, and academic rigor varies greatly, I am struck by how they all seem to focus on the infant and toddler years. If you are in need of sleep help and have graduated to eating solid foods, you're pretty much out of luck until menopause. This would not be a big deal if once your child turned three, sleep was no longer a dynamic and important aspect of their development. But your child's sleep continues to change, and it's a vital aspect of their growth. It also wouldn't be a big deal if sleep disorders in children were rare. However, of the children living in your home right now, half of them have sleep disorders, and if that statement is not true of your three kids, take pity on your neighbors who are statistically balancing out your perfect sleepers. Take this growing statistic, couple it with an inadequate system of education and treatment of pediatric sleep disorders, and you have what many experts describe as a Global Sleep Crisis in children.*

My goal for this project was to write a book to guide parents from the time their child is born and slept his first night in a crib (and before that even . . . you'll see) until they graduate high school and move out.

---

* For the remainder of this book, I am going to use the word "expert" to denote someone who is capable and qualified to study or evaluate science, specifically sleep science. Medical doctors, research PhDs, and other published individuals, many of whom are far more deserving than I am of the title "sleep expert." If you have a conspiracy-level distrust of scientists, I'm not sure this book is for you.

Crib to "crib," so to speak. This is a tough task. I know a new mother has little interest in reading about the science behind a wet dream. I also understand a frazzled father of three teenage girls who are up all night engaged in various types of social media is not interested in how to construct the best bedtime routine for a new baby.

Here is my counter—if you are the proud mother of a wonderful new baby boy, there will come a day (and it comes sooner than you think) when your son is going to mysteriously strip his bed in the morning and sheepishly offer to do his own laundry. If you understand the science behind this common occurrence heralding puberty, you are going to be better prepared for how to deal with this slightly embarrassing situation. Likewise, if you are the father of those gifted and energetic three girls, understanding how routines and activities prior to bed affect how we sleep all our lives may help you to better understand the changes that need to be made in your daughters' lives to help them have healthy sleep habits. Sleep is sleep. There really is no such thing as "Well, that really doesn't apply to me or my child."

So, organizationally, here is how this book is set up: I begin with some foundational chapters designed to get you up to speed on how sleep works. Then it is divided into sleep topics. Within each, we will examine how that topic changes and evolves through the different ages and developmental stages of a child. For some topics, like sleep need, we will discuss all different age groups of kids. For other topics of the book, like what to wear when you sleep, it is not necessary to write separately about infants and toddlers since they are both wearing the same kinds of clothes, namely items that mostly snap or zip in the crotch. Whenever possible, I'll combine various age groups to keep this show moving along at a good pace. I am going to be honest—at first, I had this book organized into developmental stages. Infants, toddlers, five- to seven-year-olds, etc. It quickly became an impossible book to write because the overlap between stages is considerable. I didn't want to have a different "snoring" section for each age group. Sleep development cannot be broken down into tidy age-oriented categories—it is a continuum, and it is individualistic.

Although there is no book on the market that is approaching sleep in kids in this way, writing about how kids sleep is not new, and much of our current beliefs have their roots in historical views on sleep. Beliefs that permeate a culture can sometimes stick, even when the science behind the belief is proven false. For example, I still deal with older adults who feel a touch of alcohol is positive when it comes to encouraging sleep, most likely because they had a grandparent who believed a little bourbon helped to soothe the nerves and encourage rest. Are things that different than they were one hundred years ago? Are we unnecessarily complicating the sleep of our children? Do our kids truly deal with new problems that they did not deal with back in the day? How will this book be judged one hundred years from now?

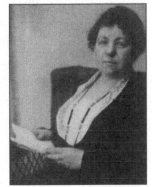

To get some perspective, and just for fun, throughout the book I've included some writing and thoughts about sleep from a leading expert in the field one hundred years ago, Anna Steese Richardson. Her book *Better Babies and Their Care* was a wealth of parental wisdom published in 1914 and one of the first to incorporate significant instructions about sleep, mentioning sleep forty-two times.*

Richardson became interested in baby health after attending a baby health contest at the National Western livestock exposition in January 1913. What's a baby health contest, you ask? Fair question. It is that thing at a county fair when babies are lined up and judged based upon "correctness of finish" and "balance/eye appeal," just like livestock. Loads of fun, with the outcome being wonderful résumé fodder for some and emotional and psychological devastation in others.†

---

* Incidentally, Samuel Ernest Bilik published *The Trainers Bible* four years later, in 1918. It was the first book believed by many to be devoted to the profession of athletic training. In it, there were twenty references to sleep. Through books like these, the growing interest in sleep and its application to health and wellness can be indirectly seen.

† "Good heavens, Matthias, he didn't even get honorable mention."

I'm a big fan of Richardson's work and how it relates to how we think about sleep in children today. However, while the book certainly means well, it does create many problematic ideas about sleep that still exist and is not afraid to blame parents for most of their baby's sleep shortcomings. Richardson did understand one very important principle about sleep: All kids do it. It is a requirement. "This is nature's warning to mothers that newborn babies need just three things: warmth, food, and sleep."* We will return to this idea of sleep as a nonnegotiable, primary need for not only a child but also for any human. This is an important concept, since many kids and their parents fear not being able to sleep. Not being able to sleep is virtually a scientific impossibility. So when you see the Anna Steese Richardson logo, you know you are getting a more historical perspective on sleep.

 So far, we have covered how this book will incorporate my modern ideas and experiences when dealing with pediatric sleep issues, and Richardson's historical-color commentary, but we do not have the voices and stories of actual patients. Fear not! I have that covered. When you see this icon, it indicates a patient story or interaction I've had with someone struggling with the topic at hand. They can tell the story far better than I can. Names have been changed, of course, for their privacy.

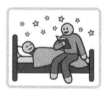 I think books about sleep are great, but I often find that there is far too much written about the science and details of a sleep disorder, and little to nothing about what can be done to help correct it. I think it's important to provide you with tools to fix these problems, so when you see this icon, it indicates an *actionable item*. In other words, here is what you can do to learn more about a disorder and ways in which to treat it. Fair warning: math may be involved.

One final thing before we get going, and it is important. While I'm

---

* Water? Oxygen?

a genuine honest-to-God neurologist and double-boarded sleep specialist who has been in the field in some way or another for twenty-eight
years, I am not someone who necessarily speaks or conducts himself in
a doctorly fashion (whatever that means) all the time. I do not wear a
white coat, and I ask my patients to call me Chris. As you're reading, imagine that you and I are sitting down somewhere quiet, enjoying a favorite
beverage, and talking about kids, sleep, and good television shows to
binge-watch, like two friends might do. Would we use words and phrases
like "hitherto," "preponderance of evidence," or "academically rigorous
evaluations have concluded"? Probably not. So if it is okay with you, I'm
going to largely avoid that kind of speak here. I'm not doing this to be
condescending. I really care about you and your kids, and I really talk
like this. So when I say something about "you and your lovely kids," I
mean it. All kids are lovely. And all kids can be great sleepers. Let's make
it happen!

And by the way, all the answers to the true/false questions were false!

The Rested Child

1

Sleep 101 for Parents

How Sleep Works in Your Kid's Brain

 Two children are sitting under my exam table fighting over an iPad featuring a virtual pet (named Lady Gaga) who requires some type of care or it will die. There is a heated disagreement as to whether it should be fed. An older girl is reading *Junie B. Jones Has a Monster Under Her Bed*, and seated next to her is Mom, who is nursing child number four.

Mom begins: "I thought I had been given the worst sleeper in the world when Emma was born, but Gabe is going to take that title from her, I think." Emma peers up from her book, looks at me with an ashamed expression, and resumes reading. Mom continues to fuss with Gabe, who truly seems to be smiling as he refuses to engage with nursing. Despite his age, it looks like he's trying to get a look at the iPad instead.

I listen and jot notes for the next twenty minutes as Mom describes a chaotic home that reminds me of the Herdmans from that book *The Best Christmas Pageant Ever*. Throughout the conversation about inconsistent sleep schedules, napping disasters, and a house that always seems to have at least one child awake and in some kind of need, Mom does not verbally leave much to the imagination when it comes to how she feels about her kids' sleep.

"They have no schedule, just like their father . . . and he wants to have another!"

~ ~ ~

There is nothing more magical than watching a baby sleep. The sight of an infant sleeping quietly, curled into roughly the position he was in when he was inside his mother's womb just days ago, is instantly sooth-ing. Watching the nuanced changes in his facial expression, the sudden muscle twitches, and subtle movements of primitive reflexes quickly re-veals to the observer that there is a wealth of changes happening inside his growing brain. As every mother or father sees their newborn sleep for the first time, a dynamic process, hidden from view, is forming the essence of who that child will be.

Prenatal Development of Sleep

As you can imagine, studying sleep in a preterm fetus is hard since it is deeply tucked away inside a lovely woman who thinks her partner is doing a lousy job rubbing her feet. Because of the technical difficulty in getting a Fitbit around an unborn baby's wrist, it is not easy to gather information on the subject. Most parents know that their baby's heart begins to beat around day twenty-two of gestation. Looking for a rela-tively simple heartbeat and measuring something as complicated as the genesis of sleeping behaviors are different beasts. Consequently, fetal sleep is a bit of a mystery to sleep researchers. Much of the data we have about the subject comes from studying animals, mainly primates. Dr. Dan Rurak, professor emeritus of maternal fetal medicine at the Univer-sity of British Columbia, noted in primate studies that sleep seems to begin at some point during the second half of gestation. In humans, as the neurological development of babies is absolutely exploding, they begin organizing their sleep into distinct patterns sometime near the beginning of the third trimester, as by then the newly formed neural network has matured to the level capable of producing this complicated process. For perhaps the first time, sleep serves as a window into the functioning of the nervous system. This reflection will be observed throughout a child's lifetime.

Neurologists are fascinated by development—the maturation of the brain, the development of neurotransmitter systems, and the behaviors that flow from them. Let's back up a little bit and examine the neurological development of a growing fetus. By week six, nerve cells begin to appear, and soon after, the brain is churning out 250,000 new cells every minute and organizing them into an intricate interconnected network. As this massive and complex system is being built, primitive rumblings of electrical activity begin to appear. Like the network itself, the early signs of sleep/wake patterns begin to emerge, and like the system as a whole, these rudimentary beginnings of sleep rapidly develop. In humans, it is thought that genuine sleep starts sometime around week twenty-seven, the beginning of the third trimester.* As this neurological network is put into place and the foundation for sleep is laid, primitive shifts of the arousal state are evident for the first time. The fetus is quiet. The fetus is kicking. For many mothers, this change is the first time this unseen, unknown life-form inside of their womb becomes real. He is in there, and he has a rhythm just like the rest of the world's inhabitants. Look who's up and busy at 3:45 a.m.!

We can see patterns of sleep and wakefulness begin to appear by halfway through the pregnancy. Usually these patterns are referred to as quiet sleep, active sleep, quiet wake, and active wake (these terms are used even though the baby is not truly ever awake). Early on, these behaviors are limited and disorganized, but as time passes, they become far more orderly and predictable. Many mothers begin to appreciate these patterns in their unborn children. While poorly studied in humans, a 2011 study on mice pups by Dr. Douglas McMahon, a pioneer in the field of chronobiology and vision, indicated that a mother's activity during

---

* This is why babies cry when they are born. They are super irritable from the twenty-seven-week all-nighter they just pulled.

the day and her circadian rhythm can influence the sleep/wake patterns of her unborn child.*

When it comes to the struggles of new parents, few are as daunting as getting a new baby to sleep. While reading some of the countless books dedicated to sleep in babies, keep in mind that "baby sleep training" (whatever that is) is happening even as a mother sits down to read a book with a baby in her belly. Mom's sleep schedule, activity level and timing, and her mealtimes may culminate in helping her unborn child begin to entrain patterns of wakefulness and rest. While research on this topic is sparse, it does exist. For example, a study in 2002 by French researchers Jean-Pierre Lecanuet and Anne-Yvonne Jacquet showed fetal heart rate response to maternal rocking (but interestingly, not gliding). Two years later, Yukari Nakajima noted a similar response with driving during pregnancy. Studies from the 1980s demonstrate relationships between maternal heart rate during sleep and that of the fetus.

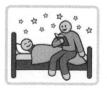 As you can imagine, the study of the relationship be-tween the behavior of a mother and the sleep of her unborn child is difficult and invasive, but there is evi-dence that the fetus has the ability to take in informa-tion and for that information to influence behavior, including the behavior of a child's sleep. Fear not, the study and under-standing of sleep will become much more accessible once the baby is born. If you happen to be pregnant and reading this book, think about the activities in which you engage every day. Sitting quietly scrolling on your phone or working at your desk, driving, exercising, eating, sleep-ing, and, of course, rocking.† Try to organize your day in such a way that these activities are happening at specific times every day. In other words, they are scheduled. For example:

* University of Virginia graduate (Wahoowa!) and disciple of Dr. Gene Block, a leg-endary circadian researcher. #RealDeal.

† Not gliding! Only rocking! We're not savages.

Up at 7:00 a.m.
Breakfast at 7:30 a.m.
Walk the dog
Quietly work for a few hours
Lunch at 12:30 p.m.
Read the paper and quietly rock for thirty minutes
More work
Cycle class
Dinner
Quiet evening and bed at 10:00 p.m.

Keep a consistent schedule full of cues so your developing baby can set the stage for better sleep well before they enter the world!

Development of Sleep in a Newborn

The baby is born.

For the first time, we can lay eyes on this rascal. Most important for sleep doctors and researchers, we finally get to observe and examine a child's sleep. In the past decade, there has been an explosion of sleep technology available to consumers. The sleep reports of these bracelets, rings, and headbands are providing more understanding about sleep terminology and sleep stages within the general population. Terms like "deep sleep" and "dream sleep" are fairly ubiquitous, and ways you can improve your own sleep are found in the pages of virtually every issue of *Men's Health, Shape, GQ,* and *Real Simple.* This is great because it gives us all a common language with which to discuss the maturing sleep of newborn babies or the sleep of a teenager. In other words, I bet you already know some things about deep sleep or have read about certain medications and their effects on sleep. While this knowledge will be very helpful (but not necessary), in newborns and infants, sleep physiology and even sleep stages are completely unique due to the relative immaturity of their brains. In addition, the amount of time it takes to move through these patterns of sleep (sleep cycles) is shorter despite their overall longer time sleeping.

Newborn babies sleep a ton and are widely considered to be the laziest and most unproductive age demographic. I made that part up, but given that some babies sleep up to eighteen hours a day, the comment feels justified. Prior to about three months old, conventional classifications of sleep are not possible since the brain has not matured enough to develop the electrical markers we look for to signify the various sleep stages.

 According to our turn-of-the-century baby expert Anna Steese Richardson, a baby will sleep twenty-two hours a day, assuming he is well taken care of. Richardson advises against family members "hanging around the crib waiting for him to wake up" and subsequently playing with him when he does awaken. "He has no desire to be moved, let alone played with."*

While I can appreciate wanting to be left alone, I'm not sure this advice has held up entirely. Most experts agree that term newborns are going to sleep seventeen to nineteen hours. Twenty-two is probably a bit too much.

Additionally, their brain's circadian rhythm is not fully formed. Think of the circadian rhythm for now as the director of programming for the Food Network. You've got twenty-four hours of television programming to fill on your cable channel and only one Bobby Flay. What are you going to do? You've got to intelligently schedule your shows for the right audience that is watching your network at any given time. How much Giada is too much Giada?† So many variables to consider. For a baby, their sleep is initially "programmed" very poorly, making the timing of their rest (and every other bodily process) inconsistent. As the child matures, this master-timing process in the brain typically does as well. Imagine the chaos and problems that arise when the circadian rhythm does not mature and develop properly, or not at all. We will revisit the circadian system in relationship to the disorders that can arise when it does not mature properly in chapter 8.

* Her descriptions of the baby always remind me of the grumpy little Monopoly man.

† Trick question: you can never have too much Giada.

Generally, newborn sleep periods average two to four hours and tend to occur around periods of feeding. This linkage of feeding times to sleep, along with light exposure, help to entrain the circadian rhythm and stabilize sleep. While this process might get its start in the newborn phase, it will stay with your child all her life, with healthy eating and light exposure playing a lifelong role in the maintenance of healthy and consistent sleep.

One variable that plays a major role in the establishment of sleep in children is the sound of their mother's voice. While babies are typically exposed to the sound of their mother speaking throughout pregnancy, the specific role it plays in soothing and sleep promotion has been unclear. Studies from the late 1980s demonstrated that a mother's voice could influence the EEG and breathing patterns in neonates. A recent study of forty-seven infants in the neonatal intensive care unit showed that babies exposed to recordings of their mothers' voices slept deeper and had fewer arousals during the night than babies who were not exposed.

"Slept deeper," "had fewer arousals" . . . what exactly is that in relation to an infant? Well, good news! Since your baby: (1) is outside the uterus, (2) has a readily accessible scalp primed for the placement of a few electrodes, and (3) cannot verbally say no, adequately control his arms, or really grab anything stuck to his scalp, we can finally get a look at what is electrically going on inside his brain while he is asleep.

Because your baby's brain is still developing and is relatively immature, during the first weeks of life, a baby's sleep differs dramatically from an adult's. In this time, this precursor to a more mature sleep is seen.* I deeply believe that parents need to be aware that this is the time when your baby is neurochemically forming the origins of its sleep, and this is a time that you can begin to have an impact on it! Let's dive into these changes and the sleep stages they indicate and examine how we measure and classify the stages.

* If adult sleep is *Sgt. Pepper's Lonely Hearts Club Band*, think of your baby's sleep as the band's early album *Meet the Beatles* . . . cute, but a bit less cohesive; shorter, not nearly as complex or fully formed.

Electrical Activity in the Brain

When examining a brain at the cellular level, we discover that the neurons that it contains create an unfathomably complex interconnected electric web with signals rapidly traveling in all directions. This electrical activity is easily measured using an electroencephalograph (EEG), a test in which an electrode is applied to an individual's scalp to measure electrical activity.

Imagine those wires measuring the electrical activity of a newborn baby's brain. What kinds of signals (or waves) are apparent? Before I answer that, let's look at some different waves these types of electrodes might display.

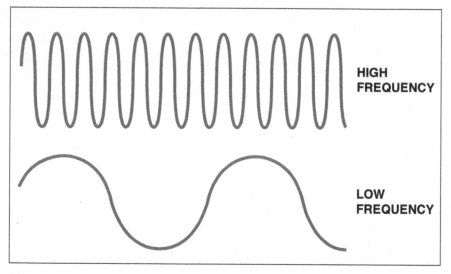

HIGH FREQUENCY

LOW FREQUENCY

Figure 1

First, think about the frequency a wave might create. Frequency relates to the number of waves one might see during a specific amount of time. In figure 1, both waves are about the same height (or amplitude), but there are twelve waves occurring on the page in the top example, but only two in the bottom example in the same period of time. Therefore, while both waves are the same amplitude, the top wave has a much higher frequency. This phenomenon is something you are probably familiar with; imagine tapping your finger on the surface of a still pool of water. Slow taps would produce a slow march of waves flowing away from your finger. Speeding up the tapping would produce a much faster wave frequency.

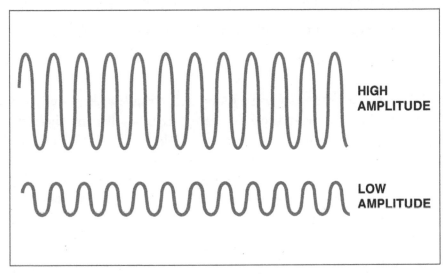

Figure 2

Amplitude is the other characteristic we often use to describe a wave. Think of it as the height of the wave. In figure 2, both the top and bottom waves have about the same frequency (twelve waves across the page), but the height, or amplitude of the top wave is about twice that of the bottom wave.

High frequency sound waves produce sounds with a higher pitch (piccolo) than low-frequency sound waves (bassoon). Conversely, high-amplitude sound waves are loud or have higher volume (a guitar with an amplifier turned up to eleven), while low-amplitude sound waves (the same amp turned down to two) are quieter.

How does this relate to sleep? Well, in the measurement of sleep, we examine waves. These waves are not produced by instruments but, in this case, the brain. Using electrodes typically applied to the scalp, these electrical waves can be recorded and studied to determine the electrical state of a brain.

If you look at a baby's brain waves long enough, distinct patterns and signatures start to emerge. With these patterns, the newborn baby's sleep is divided into the following stages:

- active sleep (a pattern similar to REM [dream] sleep);

- quiet sleep (a pattern similar to non-REM [light/deep] sleep);

- indeterminate sleep.

While it is not necessary to rush out and schedule a sleep study for your baby, there is a ton of value in looking at studies that already exist. The changes we can see in a baby's brain's electrical development are reflected in a baby's general neurological development.

Let's take a look at some newborn baby brain waves. In the following examples, what differences do you see in frequency and amplitude in the various waves?

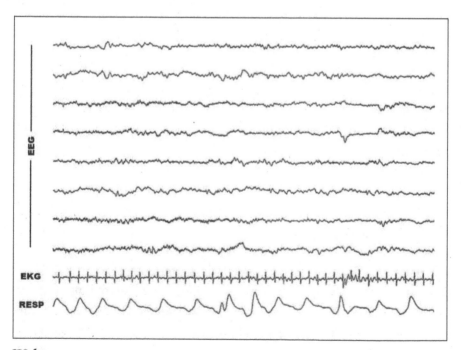

Wake

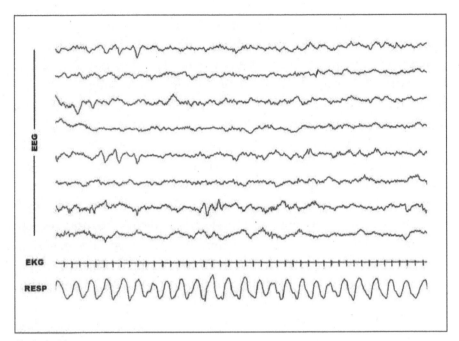

Active Sleep

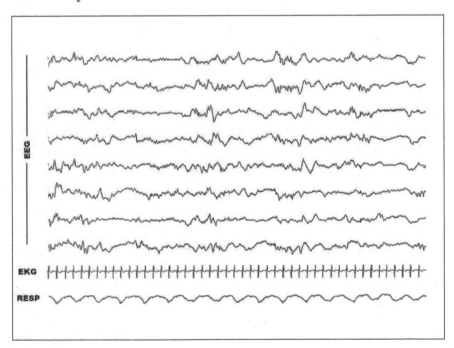

Quiet Sleep

For the first six months of a baby's life, it is pretty easy to pick out these stages of sleep behaviorally just by observing her sleep. Quiet sleep is literally just that: quiet sleep. Super boring. The baby just sits there in her carrier . . . sleeping. No moving, just rhythmic breathing. Yawn. This is usually the state babies are in when you have friends and family over and desperately want your child to perform for everyone.

Contrast this with active sleep. Ooh, now we're talking. We have little cute sucking movements, wry grins, concentrated faces, a random left arm jab—all in all it's quite a show. It is not uncommon for your mother-in-law to notice these actions and remark, "Oh, look, he's dreaming," and she's not entirely wrong, as active sleep is a precursor to dream sleep.

At birth, newborns spend equal time in both stages and generally enter into sleep via active sleep. They will spend roughly an hour in each stage, cycling back and forth between active and quiet sleep for the duration of the sleep period.

As newborns mature over that first six-month period, their sporadic 50 percent active sleep/50 percent quiet sleep architecture starts to rapidly evolve toward a more consolidated, adult-looking sleep pattern. By six months, babies begin to display patterns that look similar to adults'.* Gone are the pseudo REM and non-REM stages as the baby begins the move toward more mature stages of true REM sleep. Around this time, they will begin to split their non-REM quiet sleep into light sleep (referred to as N1 or N2 sleep) and deep sleep (N3 sleep). Additionally, during this time the baby adopts the more adult-like pattern of entering sleep via light sleep rather than during active or REM sleep. This coincides with the sleep period adding not only more cycles (equating to longer sleep periods) but also more stable sleep cycles exhibiting less interruptions. For the next several years, babies will continue on this path of consolidating their nocturnal sleep and slowly let go of daytime napping in favor of endless questions about fire engines, unicorns, and dinosaurs.

* Even at this age, they are already growing up too fast.

How Much Sleep Does My Child Need?

A question that seems appropriate at this point in the book—how much of this rapidly changing sleep does my baby need? When I meet the other parents at the park, Gio says his baby sleeps fourteen hours and Pete says his little girl sleeps much more. It's incredibly confusing—and don't get me started on comparing naps.

Let's jump into this big question right away. How much sleep does my baby need? It is a valid question, because the answer does impact everything: your baby's sleep schedule, your other kid's schedule, your schedule for getting things accomplished during the day, and arguably most important, your own sleep schedule.

National Sleep Foundation Recommended Hours of Sleep		
Age	Recommended	May Be Appropriate
Newborn (0–3 months)	14–17 hours	11–19 hours
Infant (4–11 months)	12–15 hours	10–18 hours
Toddler (1–2 years)	11–14 hours	9–16 hours
Preschool (3–5 years)	10–13 hours	8–14 hours
School Age (6–13 years)	9–11 hours	7–11 hours
Teen (14–17 years)	8–10 hours	7–11 hours
Young Adult (18–25 years)	7–9 hours	6–11 hours

Hirshkowitz, M., Whiton, K., Albert, S. M., Alessi, C., Bruni, O., DonCarlos, L., Hazen, N., Herman, J., Katz, E. S., Kheirandish-Gozal, L., Neubauer, D. N., O'Donnell, A. E., Ohayon, M., Peever, J., Rawding, R., Sachdeva, R. C., Setters, B., Vitiello, M. V., Ware, J. C., & Adams Hillard, P. J. (2015). National Sleep Foundation's sleep time duration recommendations: methodology and results summary. *Sleep health*, *1*(1), 40–43.

For newborns (zero to three months old), the National Sleep Foundation (NSF) recommends fourteen to seventeen hours of sleep per day (per twenty-four hours—in other words, include all sleep acquired in a twenty-four-hour period). The NSF goes a step further and acknowledges that there are babies who are exceptional in terms of their sleep needs and may need more or less than the "recommended" times. For these babies, they may need as much as eighteen to nineteen hours of sleep, or as few as eleven to thirteen hours.

Think about all the newborns lined up in a hospital nursery—swaddled like overstuffed Chipotle burritos. If we could see their individual sleep needs printed on their little clear rolling bassinets, we would see some of those babies with nineteen hours indicated, and others with eleven hours. That's a difference of eight hours.

What exactly accounts for such a wide variation in sleep need? The answer is pretty simple when you think about what accounts for the differences in their eye color, size, hair characteristics, and whether their earlobes are attached or dangle. Sleep need is genetic; it is inherited from their parents and is rooted in their DNA. Consequently, it varies from one baby to the next, just like their eye color.

Consider now the implications of such a wide variation in sleep need. Eight hours is *a full adult workday minus lunch!* Knowing nothing else about these nursery babies and the fine caregivers taking them home, imagine the different lives these two families are going to lead. Think about the family of the nineteen-hour baby (we can call him Lars). Wow, what a terrific sleeper Lars is! Imagine meeting his mom for lunch as she tells you how quickly he began sleeping through the night . . . how his naps are regular, prolonged affairs. Dive deeper, listen to all the things this woman is getting accomplished in her life—clean house, online MBA classes, exercise, totally caught up on *Outlander* . . .

Now, let's focus on the eleven-hour sleeper. Her name is Corta, and you just happen to run into her mom as you are leaving lunch. Ouch—different story. Corta's mom looks fried. "She is the worst—worst sleeper. . . . She never sleeps." The stories of failed naps, early-morning awakenings and desperate struggles for both child and mom to get some rest hit you so hard you are already madly looking for an exit strategy from this conversation. The lives of these two children and parents could not be more disparate.

Think about the stress levels in the homes and the language these children are going to be exposed to . . . not just tonight, but over the next several years. While Lars will be praised both directly and indirectly for his ability to sleep, Corta's sleep will be discussed in not-so-glowing terms—often within earshot of Corta herself. "She's always been a bad sleeper." "All my other kids were great sleepers; I'm not sure where we went wrong." As Corta grows up hearing these comments and feeling the stress surrounding bedtime, there is an excellent chance that she will internalize these comments as being the truth. *The seeds of sleep identity are planted when our kids are very young.* Corta is very much in danger of identifying herself as a bad sleeper and not someone who simply needs less sleep.

Big difference!

Sleep Fragmentation, Consolidation, and "Sleeping Through the Night"

Unfortunately, figuring out how much sleep a child needs is not easy. Unlike a basil plant, they don't come with that handy plastic card that tells a gardener exactly how much sunlight and water the plant requires.

The inherent fragmentation of their sleep cycles also makes it tough to get a precise feel for how much sleep they require. As the baby matures, these little pieces of sleep start to come together to form a more continuous night. This is called "sleep consolidation." It occurs most rapidly during the first four months of a baby's life. As this consolidation of sleep is happening during the night, overall total sleep time in a twenty-four-hour period is lessened.

In a 2010 study, Jacqueline Henderson, a developmental sleep researcher at the University of Canterbury, showed that depending on the definition of "sleeping through the night" one uses, babies usually hit that mark somewhere between three and six months, with two-thirds of babies sleeping through the night by six months. This is mainly a function of weight and metabolism. A baby needs to reach a weight of about twelve pounds for this magical event to happen. Achieving this milestone is an indirect indication that the baby is acquiring enough energy storage in the body to sleep through the night without getting hungry.

So far we have covered how sleep develops and evolves in a normal child. Imagine problems in these processes and how they might manifest in a baby's sleep or more general behavior. With the concept of sleep amount or sleep need, we now have a measurable variable that can give a clue as to the sleep health of your child. For parents (and sleep doctors), understanding healthy sleep and normal values and ranges can help differentiate between a child who is sleeping too much, too little, or is just right.

Understanding Sleep Consistency

In addition to sleep amount, *sleep consistency* is another important sleep variable. It is easy to miss this important factor if too much emphasis is placed on sleep amount, and a baby who sleeps the perfect *amount* every night can still have a significant sleep disorder if the *consistency* is impaired. Consider the following illustration:

As we mentioned, a baby should be getting somewhere around eleven to nineteen hours of sleep. Let's imagine that we have two babies who each require sixteen hours of sleep per day. The first baby is Jamal, and here is his sleep pattern:

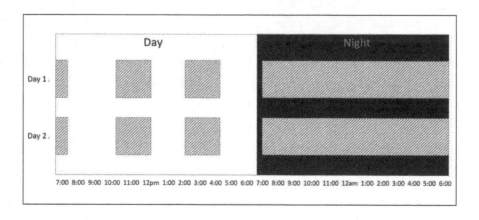

Jamal is a good sleeper according to his fathers. He goes down around 7:00 p.m. and sleeps solidly for twelve hours, awakening just as his parents are grinding the beans for their morning coffee. He usually takes two predictable naps during the day. So while his sleep is still fragmented into three sleep periods, Jamal's sixteen hours of sleep is *consistent* from one twenty-four-hour period to the next.

Contrast Jamal with another baby who sleeps sixteen hours. His name is Frankie.

As you can see, Frankie is a hot mess, rivaled only by his parents, who consider completing the most basic tasks of their own personal hygiene to be huge daily accomplishments. Frankie is killing it in terms of getting his sixteen hours, but nobody is celebrating. His sleep is fragmented

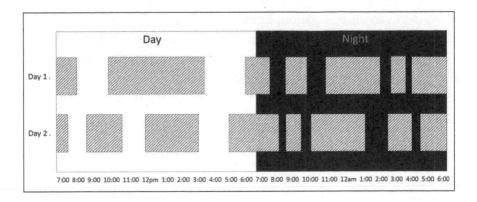

and inconsistent over the two days shown. Even Frankie himself is not thriving, despite checking the box for "sleep amount." In this example, and after spending ten minutes with Frankie and his family, it is clear that total sleep amount, all by itself, is not enough to prevent the development of a "lil' stinker."

This is probably not surprising to you. If you've ever had a night punctuated by numerous awakenings, you will appreciate the feeling. I know that when I was a doctor in training, we would get a fair amount of sleep on call. However, the broken nature of the sleep left us all feeling completely wrecked.

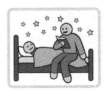

Addressing Disorders of Sleep Consistency

This early in the process, it's appropriate to take a look at your child in a very global sense. His sleep is not great, and you are going to work to improve it. At this point, we can identify some concrete sleep characteristics and use them to create strategies that we can apply to an infant, elementary student, or college freshman.

First, let's ask some preliminary questions. How much is your child sleeping within a twenty-four-hour period? Is it within normal amounts for their age group? Now, think about your child's patterns of sleep. How continuous is their sleep? Is it predictable?

If your child is having a hard time falling asleep or staying asleep, it may require some investigation. That is precisely what I want you to do now: begin the investigation. Look over this list of potential obstacles that might be preventing your child from getting the full amount of sleep they need or preventing adequate continuity. Do you believe any of these issues or conditions are in play?

reflux
colic
pain
hunger
diaper rash
electronics
abnormal eating patterns
noise in the home
outside environmental noise
disruption from a sibling
pets
light in the bedroom

There are a couple of points to this exercise. First, it is a first step into the world of pediatric sleep hygiene. You are making sure that the stage is properly set for your child to sleep effectively. Second, you are taking care to control the things under your control so that if you see a sleep specialist in the future, you are prepared to report on the multiple potential sleep disruptors that you will invariably be asked about. Remember, much of the art of medicine and diagnosis is like a game of twenty questions!

 "You are giving Lady Gaga too much food. Stoooooooo oooop."

Before I even open the exam room door or take a peek at the chart, I know exactly which family awaits inside my exam room. It appears Emma, Gabe, Mom, and the rest of the crew have returned, and there is a noticeably more upbeat feel in the room.

Mom begins. "Things are a lot better. Emma has been doing great.

We are letting her stay up and read in her room at night, and that has made a big difference. We were putting all the kids to bed at the same time because, frankly, I just needed a break. I think you were right. We were just expecting too much sleep from Emma. Even Gabe's schedule, once I added it all up, had him sleeping eighteen hours. He seems much more suited for sixteen. I always thought that you should just let the kids tell you when they want to sleep, but since trying to make his days a little more consistent, it has really changed the way he sleeps. He's a good sleeper now."

"I'll bet he was always a good sleeper. Most kids are, they just need some direction here and there," I replied.

"Ahhhhhhhhhhhhhhh! See, I told you that was too much food," screamed a voice from underneath the exam table. "Now Lady Gaga is sick and is pooping everywhere."

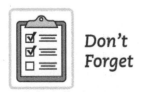 **Don't Forget**

1. Sleep appears in your unborn baby sometime in the third trimester. This is a great time to start thinking about how your behaviors will influence her sleep.

2. Your baby's sleep is going to change quickly and dramatically.

3. Keep in mind that your baby's sleep need may be very different from those of other children his age.

4. Always think about consistency as you monitor your child's sleep schedule.

2

Sleep Beliefs

Your Parents Were Wrong About Everything,
from Pills to Naps to Cosleeping.

There are certain magical questions in my clinic. One of them is, "What time does your child nap?" There is a direct relationship between the time it takes a parent to answer that question and the health of their child's sleep. In this example, I asked Jackson's mom that question. Here is her answer, which may as well have been a PowerPoint presentation:

"Well, it all depends on Jackson's sleep last night and what I'm doing that day. If I have to volunteer at Books for Babies, he won't get his nap until after lunch, unless I'm on sorting duty instead of distribution duty. If I'm on sorting duty, he will sometimes lay down on this couch we have in the office and sleep. If I'm doing distribution, he is with me in the car and he won't sleep. On those days, he will sleep for over an hour when we get home, if his dad is working. If Dad is home, forget about it. Jackson is way too interested in the car he's rebuilding in the garage. He lets Jackson help."

The story goes on and on, yet when it's time for me to dictate the encounter, I have virtually nothing to say except for, "Jackson is a three-year-old who is struggling with sleep, in particular his napping regularity. Jackson has no nap schedule."

~ ~ ~

Science, science, science. I know there were a lot of pictures of the brain's electrical activity in that first chapter, but it is absolutely necessary for you to have at least a glimpse into the workings of *how* your child sleeps. When I was younger, my dad would always try to get me interested in *how* an engine ran or *how* to clean a fish you've caught. At the time, I was more interested in *how* to become a spy or *how* to receive quality ninja training.

With the *how* out of the way, it is time to move on to four more basic questions that confront parents of all ages:

Who is your child in terms of their sleep identity?

Where should a child sleep?

When should a child sleep?

What do I give my child who struggles to sleep?

The Mythology of Sleep

Before we dive into these topics, it is worth mentioning why I grouped them all together and put them early in the book. The simple answer lies in a side of sleep I find absolutely fascinating: the mythology of sleep. Despite all of the science, theory, and research that surrounds sleep, the things you've heard about sleep during your lifetime—little sayings, stories, remedies, tales, assumptions—play a profoundly important role in a child's sleep development. Remember this little terrifying fact from any sleepover you attended in middle school? "If you die in your sleep, you die in real life." WHAT? And sticking with the slumber party theme, remember the highly scientific studies you and your friends conducted on the first partygoer to fall asleep—taking their hand and putting it in warm water to see if they would wet their sleeping bag? Classic. So, what do these topics have in common? They are themes that are central to stories and legends of the shadowy history and science of sleep. Often rooted loosely in fact, these sleep myths are both fascinating and instructive topics to explore.

"Want to keep bad dreams away? Sleep with a knife, fork, and spoon under your pillow." As your kid matures, myriad tips and bits of advice like these are everywhere.* While medicine in general seems to attract its own kind of parallel lore, sleep specifically is a hotbed of these kinds of stories. As a parent today where everyone has an opinion on Facebook, it is important to separate out what is real and what is not.

This section will explore parental beliefs about sleep, how babies/children/teens sleep, the unique properties of their sleep, and how parental behavior influences the development of healthy sleep in children. As you read this section and think about the way we talk and discuss sleep, I want you to pay particular attention to how these topics might influence the way a child begins to internalize ideas and beliefs about sleep—in particular how well she sleeps. These experiences and dialogues with you will help to form her sleep identity, and this sleep identity will play an enormous role in determining her relationship with sleep over her entire lifetime.

Sleep Identity

Without a doubt, sleep identity is one of the biggest myths that circulates within parent culture. Almost immediately after a child is born, we begin to label and assign values. In my experience, some of the first include (please check only one):

WEIGHT

❐ Big boy

❐ Little guy

ACTIVITY

❐ So interested in everything

❐ Serious

---

* Seriously, the silverware under the pillow is a real comment several patients have made!

NURSING

❏ Hungry little fella

❏ Too curious to eat right now

SLEEP

❏ A champion sleeper like Granddad

❏ Bad sleeper like Grandma

And just like that, the race for identity formation is on. Initially, this identity is the sole projection of her parents, family, and friends, as most newborns do not declare themselves to be fundamentally opposed to a foreign-policy position stressing globalization or to consider thin-crust pizza to be a culinary abomination.

"Wow, you are such a healthy eater—future linebacker!"
"Look how smart she is. . . . She just loves to explore and see things."
"When he looks at the television and drools, who does he remind you of?
"Oh my, when she walks, you can tell she's going to be a little ballerina!"
"She is such a fussy sleeper."

The sleep-identity phenomenon has been the subject of several scientific studies, and the results are surprising. In many cases, how an individual *actually* sleeps takes a secondary role to how an individual *thinks* he sleeps. In other words, a child's belief that she is a good sleeper often has a significant impact on how that child approaches sleeping or how she feels in the morning and often throughout the following day. Additionally, I often see adult patients pointing to their childhood sleep as evidence that they're "bad sleepers" now—as if their adult sleep habits are rooted in how they slept when they wore a diaper and cried anytime somebody made their face disappear with their hands. This is not only a self-limited sleep crisis of children, but left untreated, the problems amplify over time to contribute to the sleep epidemic we have in adults as well.

Generally, this sleep identity is summed up by one sentence. It pains me when I hear it in my clinic. It is definitive yet vague; seemingly simple yet strangely complex. It is usually the first thing out of a parent's mouth when I enter the exam room and see parent and child sitting there fighting over the iPad.

My child is a *bad* sleeper.

Bad sleeper? Really? I am rarely introduced to kids who are "bad students." Kids "struggle" in school. They are not bad at school. Kids are "having some trouble making friends," they are not bad friends. Kids who have weight issues are not "bad at being thin." Why, then, with the kids sitting right there in the room, do we say that they are bad sleepers?

The short answer probably lies in the idea that many parents have decided that their child's sleep ability is sort of like their eye color: genetic and therefore outside their control. They see their friend's child (Lars!) and his uncanny ability to sleep perfectly as a God-given gift.*

Sleep ability is not outside of your control. We are talking about a kid who takes a while to fall asleep. Maybe it is a kid who wakes up in the night and wants water. Maybe this bad sleeper is a child who comes into her parents' room and wakes them up. At any rate, it is important to ask a simple but tough question: What's really bad here? Your child's behavior, or how your child's behavior is meeting your expectations and influencing your life?

These issues start early, with most developmental researchers believing that the main determinant of a child's identity and ego come from those closest around her. Like a little sponge, she is absorbing information, behaviors, and small cues constantly. Children watch what you do. They hear what you say. This is not new information. Research has clearly shown that anxiety is often "caught" from parents who display

---

* While sleep amount is genetically influenced, sleep amount and sleep ability are not the same thing!

anxious tendencies. Mechanisms proposed in this type of transmission can easily be applied to sleep disorders.

These mechanisms of parent-child transference include these three things:

1. **Fatalistic mirroring:** Sleep disorders and the anxiety about sleep disorders in parents are transmitted to children. In other words, a parent's disproportionately negative response to a bad night of sleep would be seen by a child and eventually imitated.

> **Negative:** "I had a terrible night last night and now I feel awful. I can't go to work today."

> **Positive:** "That was a difficult night. I'm sure that with a good breakfast and maybe a latte today I can charge through this day, hit the gym after work, and be fine tomorrow."

2. **Aberrant response:** Sleep disorders create negative parenting pathways that either cause or reinforce poor sleep in their children. The stressful feedback at bedtime or during the night often works to increase a child's anxiety about their own sleep, worsening the problem. Parents who struggle with sleep disturbances frequently regard themselves as being functionally impaired or completely dysfunctional.* Nevertheless, this impairment, whether real or perceived, can impact the skills necessary for them to effectively parent. Ineffective parenting techniques (losing patience, getting upset with a child for coming out of his room, etc.) can itself lead to increased anxiety about sleep in their children.†

---

* "Completely dysfunctional" is a curious term, since they have obviously woken up, dressed themselves, operated their smartphone, navigated to my office, and recalled their entire life's sleep history for me. To me, that seems pretty functional.

† Speaking of losing patience, I remember taking care of my newborn son during my first year of neurology residency. As I was about to go into his room to deal with his

Negative: An exhausted parent with disabling chronic pain screams at her child, "There are no monsters under your bed, but if you come out of that room one more time to have me check for them, I'll find one and put it there."

Positive: A mother in the midst of a fibromyalgia flare recognizes the influence her pain has on her parenting skills in the moment and defers to her partner to help with her children until her pain is under better control. In situations where that is not viable, Mom acts with honesty: "Mom loves you but is in too much pain to keep checking under your bed for imaginary monsters. You are going to be fine. Please help me feel better by staying in your room if you can."

3. **Negative reinforcement:** In children, sleep issues themselves can quickly begin to influence the parenting interventions they receive. In other words, their sleep behaviors may influence the way in which we parent, turning a small benign problem into a much more metastatic one.

Negative: Allowing a child to sleep in bed with you, have a TV in their bedroom to help them "relax," or allowing an older child to nap throughout the day after a difficult night.

Positive: Making sure parental interventions are geared toward a more positive long-term sleep outcome and not a convenient temporary fix. These might include waking a child up on time to maintain a schedule, not giving in to letting them have an iPad in their bed, etc.

Let's look at an example of how all of these scenarios could play out. Recently, I spoke to a woman with a lifelong history of sleep problems and anxiety. When I asked her about the start of her sleep problems, she

---

endless crying, I angrily called my two-month-old "an idiot." After saying it I froze and looked at my wife in horror. Then we both laughed hysterically and walked into the bedroom.

immediately pointed to childhood. The daughter of a mother who was a nurse and a military-officer father, she was often sharply reprimanded for staying up and reading in bed when she could not fall asleep. Over time, fear of being discovered in bed awake by her father resulted in many abnormal behaviors and fears surrounding her bedtime and sleep.

Here we have a child who is simply being asked to go to bed a little too early. She's attempting to sleep when she is not particularly sleepy. That's it. That is the entire problem in its most fundamental form. Her parents are telling her to go to sleep earlier than she is able. Thinking about her parents' careers (nurse, military officer), one might guess that they are relatively *short sleepers*—individuals who genetically require a little less sleep than the average individual. Short sleepers thrive in business, medical, and military occupations, as sleep is often at a premium and not always readily available. Often, short sleepers not only fail to recognize themselves as such but also fail to recognize that they have passed this trait onto their children. In other words, their eight-year-old does not need the same amount of sleep as all the other eight-year-olds in the neighborhood.

Without this critical piece of information, parents of short sleepers often expect their children to sleep as much as other kids—but they don't, and they can't. It is literally not in their genes! So this child has a minor sleep issue that will soon influence the way her parents interact with her. As you can imagine, Father may interpret the failure of his daughter to sleep as "not following the rules." His own sleep deprivation that goes along with a high leadership post creates impatience and explosive bouts of anger when he sees the light on in his daughter's bedroom late at night (**aberrant response**), which can create terrific anxiety in his daughter when she hears him coming up the stairs toward her room. Concurrently, Mom is worried and frequently warns her daughter that if she does not go to sleep, she will get sick and do poorly in school (**fatalistic mirroring**). As time passes, the worsening of her sleep and her growing fear/dread of being in bed leads to napping after school and prolonged sleep on weekends (**negative reinforcement**). With the situation getting worse, her parents' fears about her sleep (**fatalistic mirroring**) and their capacity for effective parenting (**aberrant response**) sum to establish a truly damaging downward spiral, eventually resulting in an adult who has spent decades on sleeping pills (perhaps the ultimate in **negative reinforcement**) and introduces herself as "the worst sleeper you'll ever see, Doc."*

A lifetime of sleep torment and strife develops solely because genetically, as an eight-year-old, this woman needed eight hours of sleep (instead of ten) and should have been going to bed at 10:00 p.m. instead of being put in bed with the lights out at 8:00 p.m.

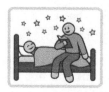

Cultivating a Positive Sleep Outlook

In the same way you consider your words and behaviors as they relate to your son's body image or daughter's concerns over poor grades in math, consider the feedback you are giving them about their sleep and the portrayal of your own sleep issues, if they exist. Work on cultivating a positive and confident sleep outlook for your child by praising a positive night of sleep, and helping to appropriately frame a more difficult night. It is widely known that a big problem evident in individuals with sleep disorders is a tendency to dwell on a small number of problematic nights and completely disregard a vast majority of good nights. Let your child know that it is not only common, but completely normal, to have a difficult time sleeping from time to time. Sometimes we are hungry for lunch, other times we are not. We are taught that appetite can fluctuate. Sleep drive can do the same thing.

When a child wants to talk about their difficult night, it is good to listen and allow them to express their thoughts, anxieties, and stress about the situation. Let your words temper the negative feelings, not amplify them. Instead of "Ugh, your sleep last night sounds terrible. I hope you don't have another bad night tonight when you try to sleep. I'm afraid if it keeps happening, you'll get sick, miss school, and fall behind." Wow, it sounds like your seven-year-old's college options are on the line based upon how quickly they'll fall asleep tonight. A better way to phrase your response might be: "I'm sorry you had a bad night, but they happen

* This is an actual example of a woman I saw in my practice, and she really said that.

to everyone, even the best sleepers. Fortunately, your body is built to do just fine after a night of bad sleep, especially when most of your nights are as awesome as yours. I bet your body will sleep extra well tonight to make up for it. Let's go eat some breakfast." *Acknowledge* the night, *recontextualize* the night as something your body considers to be relatively normal, and finally *reassure* your child that his body can handle it, and that most of his nights are perfectly fine. End on a note that inspires confidence and optimism, not fear. I promise if you can make this a habit, you will save him a visit to my office in thirty years!

Cosleeping

Let's go back in time to a cave somewhere. Our more primitive ancestors are gathered around a fire and sleeping huddled together to conserve body heat. There are no beds, no individual rooms, and no cameras filming and marketing the event as a reality television experience titled *Naked and Afraid*.*

Today, sleep in various parts of the world looks very dissimilar from that primitive sleeping arrangement. Culturally and historically, children's sleeping environments are dramatically different depending on where you are reading this book right now.

It is important to note that just because something has changed over time does not make it bad or wrong. Sure, we used to sleep piled on top of one another in a cave, I suppose, but we also used to banish people with leprosy and smoke cigarettes in operating rooms. We evolve.

 It is hard to find a topic related to the sleep of a child more inundated with myth and lore than where a child sleeps. Anna Steese Richardson says:

From birth, the baby should sleep alone in a dark room well ventilated.

---

* "Thog is not pulling his weight in our group, which is so unfair. All he does is sit around and complain. This firewood is not going to collect itself."

The baby should not be rocked to sleep, nor should he be tucked into a carriage and then trundled to sleep. In clear weather he may be snuggled up in his carriage and set out of doors in a corner screened, from draught or direct rays of the sun, for both his morning and afternoon naps. At 6 o'clock, he should be undressed, made perfectly comfortable, fed and then laid down on a firm hair mattress without a pillow, to go to sleep without further attention.

Let's defer our discussion about "hair mattresses" and why the term makes me throw up a little in my mouth. The prevailing wisdom at the turn of the century could be kindly defined as "less is more." Today, babies sleep in a variety of places: bassinets, cribs, boxes, or tucked in right beside a parent in his or her bed. For many parents, it is one of the first decisions that is made after birth. Up until that point, most kids were buzzing around the hospital like Baby Yoda in that cool bassinet on wheels with the helpful stainless-steel drawer underneath. Unfortunately, that bassinet does not come with the baby, so you can't take it home. Now you have to make a choice!*

While there was probably no guidance as to *where* the child should sleep, there was probably instruction as to what position your child should be in. "Back to sleep" is generally the preferred position for children to assume in bed, with many published studies showing that this position significantly reduces the risk of sudden infant death syndrome (SIDS). Currently, the American Academy of Pediatrics (AAP) recommends this as the preferred sleeping position for infants. The institution of this policy has cut the incidence of SIDS by half.

A quick word on SIDS. It is not rare. In 2017, it was the fourth leading cause of infant death, which includes:

1. congenital malformations (e.g., a birth defect that resulted in death), 118.8 per 100,000 births (.12 percent);

---

* Many babies today are not born in hospitals but rather at home, in birthing centers, or in the backs of Ubers. Just wanted to give you guys your props!

2. low birth weight (often too premature to live), 97.2 per 100,000 births (.097 percent);

3. maternal complications, 37.1 per 100,000 births (.037 percent);

4. SIDS 35.5 per 100,000 births (.036 percent).

While .036 percent sounds small, considering the fact that there were 3,853,472 live births in 2017, 1,368 baby deaths are not insignificant. Also consider that the reporting and classification of a death as being the result of SIDS is thought to be significantly underreported because of (1) the complexity of making the formal diagnosis and ruling out other causes, (2) the requirement that the death be labeled "SIDS" and not "asphyxia" or some other diagnosis/diagnostic code, and (3) the reluctance of some organizations, hospitals, or doctors to ever use the term "SIDS."

SIDS is not a new problem, even if the term is relatively modern. Even Richardson seems to address "crib death" more than one hundred years ago, and she does not pull any punches.

From birth, the baby should sleep alone, in a dark room well ventilated.

Bottom line with Richardson. Don't even bother entering your child into the Central Kansas Baby Health Contest if she's sleeping in bed with you. She continues:

Baby knows no fear and needs no light. Neither does he need the warmth of an adult body. There have been sad tragedies of babies smothered by tired mothers, too heavy with sleep to know they had rolled over on the tiny, helpless form. There have been other cases where babies permitted to sleep with adults, afflicted with chronic disease, have contracted the ailment and died.

So where should they sleep? Up until relatively recently, governing bodies like the AAP were reluctant to take a position on the matter.

However, after numerous studies seemed to point to cosleeping as a risk factor, alarms were sounded. The resultant recommendations of the studies are summarized here:

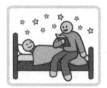 **Where Your Child Should (and Shouldn't) Sleep**
In 2016, the AAP recommended that children not sleep with their parents in the same bed but ideally rather in a bassinet or cot next to the parental bed. This should be the case for at least six months, ideally for one year. Other recommendations included:

1. Infants should be placed on their backs to sleep. This one simple action can reduce the chances of infant crib death by 50 percent.

2. Infants should sleep on a firm sleeping surface with a fitted sheet that does not indent when the child sleeps on it. Additionally, cribs should not have wide slats or missing hardware, and should conform to current government safety standards.

3. Soft objects like stuffed animals and bulky bedding should not be used. I often see cribs with elaborate bumpers and soft/luxurious bedding. This kind of bed setup is not appropriate for infants and toddlers.

4. Commercial devices used to prevent SIDS should be avoided. These include positioners or devices meant to separate the infant (sleeping with others in an adult bed) from the other sleepers.

5. Swaddling should not be utilized as a technique to prevent SIDS.

There is much more information included in the *Pediatrics* 2016 update related to sleeping safety (including supervised "tummy time" to help infants develop the ability to gain shoulder girdle strength and to avoid flattening of the back of the head from prolonged positioning in a supine position).

Diving deeper into the supporting studies that the task force utilized to draft this document, there are some additional findings that, while not in the final recommendations, are worth considering.

First, while there was clear evidence to suggest cosleeping was dangerous (either spending the entire night in bed with adults, or being brought into bed for the later part of the night, which is often the case after a nocturnal feeding, for example), there was also evidence that an infant sleeping in a room separated from her parents was at risk as well. Falling asleep on a couch with a parent also seemed to carry an increased risk.

There is a large community that supports cosleeping, and I support many aspects of their movement. If we adopt a more evolutionary perspective, the idea of sleeping apart from a child is a relatively new development. The connection a parent feels with their child at night can be very meaningful and dear. While it may disrupt parent sleep quality and foster a sleeping situation that is difficult to move away from later,* there are other potential benefits. James McKenna, an anthropologist and sleep researcher, has a book called *Safe Infant Sleep* if you want his perspective on the topic. It should be noted that his recommendations and those posted on his University of Notre Dame Mother-Baby Behavioral Sleep Laboratory, at the time of this writing, do differ from the current American Academy of Pediatrics recommendations.

There is a potential developmental downside to cosleeping as well, as research exists that suggests cosleeping children slept fewer hours, had more sleep disturbances and bedtime resistance, and had more behavioral and emotional problems than independent sleepers.

Here is my bottom line. Have you ever gone to a dinner party and seen a young woman quietly refuse the offer of red wine and then ten minutes later everyone is celebrating the exciting news of a pregnancy? Sure you have. Why did she not take a sip of alcohol? Is it because one sip of alcohol is likely to harm her unborn child? No. There is credible

---

* "Sweetie, can you take your laptop somewhere else to do your calculus homework? Daddy and I need to sleep."

evidence to support the idea that small amounts of alcohol, even early in pregnancy, do not harm the fetus or increase the risk of adverse pregnancy outcomes at all.

Why she really declined the merlot, and rightfully so, is this—she wants to control what she can control and do everything in her power to ensure a positive outcome for her pregnancy. Bad things unfortunately happen. What that mother wants to say, no matter what happens, is, "I did everything I could do for my child to ensure his health and safety." Decisions regarding an infant's sleep environment should receive the same level of care and attention.

My position on cosleeping is also personal. I know parents who have accidentally killed their child in bed, as their physician and also their friend. One of my own employees lost her five-and-a-half-month-old grandchild this way—her daughter got up early to leave for work, and her son-in-law thought the baby had been put back in the bassinet but was actually in bed with him, and the child suffocated. I can personally bear witness to the fact that the subsequent devastation and ruin it brought upon the family is something akin to a bomb going off in one's living room. In this case, the marriage quickly deteriorated, feelings of blame and regret were crippling, and substance abuse for the involved father quickly followed.

If this happened to you, would you still be happy with your decision to have your child in bed with you? I've seen mountain climbers or BASE jumpers say during interviews that if they die, it is okay with them because a life without scaling a sheer mountain face or leaping off a bridge is simply a life they do not want to live. Even distraught family members after the tragedy seem comforted by the fact that their loved one died doing something about which they were passionate. In other words, the potential price of death or disability is worth the ticket to ride. In my experience, I have yet to encounter a parent who shares that sentiment after the tragedy has unfolded. In fact, all of them expressed deep and profound regret that they had made the decision to have the child in the bed with them. In all the cases to which I have been privy, alcohol was never involved, nor were any other actions I would deem even partially negligent . . . outside of the decision to sleep with their baby. Incidentally, all vow never to do it again.

So hold your baby. Snuggle with your baby. Talk to your baby. Read to your baby. Buy your baby little onesies that have your favorite football team logo on them.* When it comes to sleeping, have them in a little safety-approved bassinet right next to your bed for at least the first year.

Napping

Decisions have been made as to where the little guy is going to lay his head at night, and perhaps with whom. Splendid. Now, when should he embark on the endeavor of sleep? Most of us can agree that the night should be a big part of his sleep routine, but what about sleeping in the day? While napping is generally thought about as a part of a baby's sleep schedule, it continues to be part of the daily schedule for kids of all ages . . . even college students.

Outside of questions about how much sleep a child or teen should get, no other topic is of more concern and worry than napping. Entire books are dedicated to elaborate nap schedules and variations based upon an inordinate number of variables that only those who have studied matrix algebra and advanced mathematical modeling could possibly understand.

When it comes to conceptualizing napping, keep things simple. Think of it as a "sleep snack," similar to the food we eat between our three meals of the day. Remember that really popular book about how to figure out what snacks to give to your kids and when to give them? Neither do I. It seems pretty straightforward. If your kid is hungry and dinner isn't for a few hours, give him some Goldfish crackers and continue living your life.†

I want you to think about napping in this way too. Simply. As we go through some thoughts and ideas about naps, the main rule here is that we keep things simple.

The first thing to be aware of with napping is that the sleep your child

---

* "Lil' Packer"

† Both hunger and sleep are considered primary drives. They are things our bodies *must* have, like water and Louis Vuitton bags. I love using food analogies as a stand-in for sleep.

gets during her nap (or naps) is real sleep. In other words, it counts. It is not some kind of extra-credit bonus sleep that does not factor into a child's daily sleep need. Remember the NSF sleep need chart from chapter 1? The heading reads "hours of sleep," not "hours of sleep at night." In other words, that number is their sleep need *per twenty-four hours*.

What that means is that just like a family-sized bag of chips can "spoil dinner," a child's two-hour nap may "spoil" nighttime sleep. It's all one big allotment. This is a concept that I am as likely to discuss with a new mother as I am a grandmother who falls asleep every afternoon watching *Hot Bench* on the couch.

For young children, this relates directly to the concepts of *sleep need* and *sleep consistency* that we have already examined. It also directly plays into the ongoing thread of *sleep identity*, because the ability to nap may be the most coveted attribute a parent could ever wish for in their child.

When it comes to napping in little ones, do not overthink it. A newborn baby can nap up to five times a day, and by the time his first birthday party happens, he'll probably be down to two. You can map them out from the start, a method favored by parents who already have older kids on a schedule, or you can play it by ear . . . taking cues from the natural patterns of your baby. Either way is fine, but regardless of the method, the plan should result in definitive nap times.

MEDICAL SCIENCE DEPARTURE ALERT

Some parents let their children nap whenever they like. This can even include letting a child sleep in an attended running car in a Whole Foods parking lot when a baby falls asleep on the way to a store. While there is ample research on the benefits of napping (a 2019 study of 3,819 elementary school students showed afternoon napping benefited the children cognitively, psychologically, and emotionally), there is little systematic research on the effects of nap timing.

So I am going to warn you that I am about to move toward an educated opinion and away from evidence-based medicine when I say that *naps should be scheduled*. In later sections of the book, you are going to see how critically important the role of biological timing and the circadian rhythm is within your child. For that reason, we want to give your baby definitive markers related to time throughout the day. In the same way I endorse a set bedtime and wake time, I also favor set nap times, understanding, of course, that this schedule can change over time as your child matures. If you want my advice, the timing of the naps you choose for your baby matters much less than making sure those times are consistent from day to day. Your baby is looking to you for help organizing its brain. The early structure you provide here will pay off big in the future in terms of your growing child's ability to sleep.

This can be tough. There are not many parents who put their child down for an hour-long nap, and when it takes their kid fifty-five minutes to fall asleep, wake them up after a five-minute snooze and go about their day. But that is exactly what a scheduled nap should look like. Moreover, any attempts made by your child to sleep outside the nap period need to be thwarted. If you want a good napper, you must make a good napper. Offer opportunities to sleep. If your child does not need or take advantage of that opportunity, then offer them another one later—on a schedule that you have created based upon observed need and/or needs of the family.

And back to science—a good napper is a healthy napper. These investments in napping pay off. Dr. Klára Horváth, a developmental psychologist, concluded in a 2018 literature review that daytime napping was essential for the development of memory. While other studies have suggested daytime napping could have a much broader reach in terms of health and cognitive benefits, the inconsistencies in the findings as well as the inconsistencies in the ages and napping patterns studied makes drawing definitive conclusions difficult.

Beyond the health benefits of napping, the mere presence and eventual disappearance of napping may have developmental meaning in your child. I remember being told that kids who lost their teeth early were smarter than those who held on longer to their baby chompers.* Emerging research is showing that the need for a nap may be a marker

---

* Or was it later teething that is the sign? Either way, I could find no credible studies linking teething or losing baby teeth and intelligence.

for cognitive development in young sleepers, with the early loss of napping potentially a sign of accelerated neurological maturation. We will address napping in teens later. For now, just keep in mind that they should not be allowed to stay up late on Snapchat or playing *Call of Duty* and then expect to nap during the day. That is not the kind of napping we are talking about here!

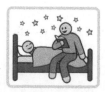

Napping 101

If we are all in agreement that naps are a good thing for kids, particularly young children under the age of five, let's establish some simple rules for making naps happen.

From the start and for your own understanding, you should not refer to the nap as a nap when talking to your kids. It is a rest. Napping implies sleep, and sleep sometimes will happen, and sometimes it will not. When you ask your child to sleep, there is a performance anxiety that he will associate with the act, and you will as well. Imagine your daughter when she is older, shooting free throws for fun on the driveway. Now imagine her at the line shooting two to win a state championship. Do you feel the anxiety as you watch from the bleachers? She feels it too. And even though it's the same action: rubber ball through iron hoop, that psychological layer we've added to the act can be crippling. To keep that from happening, we have "rest periods" during the day where the goal is simple: rest. If your child sleeps, that's great, but our stated goal is rest.

There is a big difference between sleep and rest. If I say, "One, two, three . . . go to sleep now," I'm doubtful you or any child could achieve that goal quickly. It's not completely under our moment-to-moment control. If I say, "One, two, three . . . now rest," anyone can kick off their shoes, lean back, close their eyes, and *pow*, you're resting. One hundred percent under our control.

And control is what we want to give to our children. Control of their future. Control of who they are and who they love. Control of their faith and beliefs. Control of their health and sleep. By establishing *rest* and not *sleep* as an expectation, you are essentially telling your child that they can't lose! Oh, and when it comes to the benefits of resting versus sleep, they are both exceptionally beneficial to our bodies and minds.*

Naps should end in the same way that a child's nocturnal sleep period ends: definitively. Wake your child up gently but firmly when the rest time is over. Even if they only slept for a few minutes, praise the effort. Let them know how beneficial the time was. Maybe let them know that you rested too (this is helpful on many levels, not the least of which, it keeps your kid from thinking he missed out on something fun). Immediately get them active, ideally somewhere warm, well lit. Don't let them sleep until the next nap.

Finally, napping is reserved for efficient sleepers. What I mean by this is if your child is struggling with sleep continuity at night, the napping schedule during the day may need to be reevaluated. A common sign of maturity and corresponding decline in sleep need is a new increase in nocturnal sleep fragmentation. When a child is having issues falling or staying asleep at night, that is often a sign that the brain is indicating the presence of *too much sleep opportunity and not enough sleep motivation.* This is a good time to consider shaving off fifteen to thirty minutes from a daytime nap opportunity. As kids mature, the nocturnal sleep period can be reduced as well, but generally naps go before nighttime sleep goes, given the ultimate goal of a consolidated period of nocturnal sleep.

In some families, particularly with multiple children, there is a "family rest time" in which all the kids have a rest period. Our kids kept a rest time on their schedule until their later elementary years, and I'll admit, it was as much for Mom and Dad as it was for their memory development. With no electronics allowed, sometimes they slept, often they read or drew, and we had a chance to recharge our own batteries so we could be better parents. Having an eye on the development of such a period can be useful as you decide what rest periods to drop as your kids mature.

Finally, a word of caution about napping. If your child suddenly reverts back to needing more sleep or napping excessively, don't ignore this

---

* This is precisely why one of the frequent sayings in our clinic is "Do not judge success or failure in bed by unconsciousness."

sign. Conditions causing hypersomnia (many covered later in this book) may often first announce their arrival by a new tendency for a child who has never napped to suddenly nap constantly. While staying up too late is often the default explanation, it is not in some kids. Trust your gut if you think something is wrong, and talk to your child's primary care doctor about your concerns. Remember, children should need less sleep as they mature, not suddenly need more. This is a trend that will continue their entire lives.

Sleep Remedies and Sleeping Pills

Parents care about the health and well-being of their children, yet outside of how a child generally looks, behaves, eats, and sleeps, there are not many easy ways for parents to get a look inside their kid's health. This is probably why we are so strangely hung up on sleep if it's not working as we think it should.

To the extent that we feel best when we have control over things, we all want to control the health of our kids and their sleep. One way to do that is with medicine. It's good for what ails you, and it has been for a long time, with sleep potions and elixirs dating back probably to the dawn of recorded history.

At some point, you have probably been recommended something for sleep. While pills are all the rage today, remedies were often relied upon on to get your great-grandfather to sleep when he was a baby. Whiskey with honey, honey and whiskey, a spoonful of honey dipped in whiskey, and honey-free whiskey were quite the rage. Vintage magazines contain advertisements for drugs that were specifically aimed at helping kids sleep. My favorite is Pabst Extract made by the fine people who have brought you Pabst Blue Ribbon beer (so named for all the awards their beers began winning as far back as 1876). Pabst Extract was essentially malt liquor (the ingredients were not listed in the labeling or advertisements), and while it was not overtly advertised as something to give your wound-up children, many stories exist of children receiving a slug when sleep was an issue. Incidentally, for Anna Steese Richardson, her favorite was "broth or gruel as a sleep coaxer."

This begs the question—what constitutes a sleep issue necessitating medicinal intervention? Most of the time, the child's sleep problem looks pretty similar to ours today—a child having trouble falling asleep, or perhaps a teenager who awakens and cannot return to sleep. What's the big deal?

In the past, the big deal was twofold. First, the inability to provide your child with proper rest is inextricably linked to notions of parental guilt. You were a bad parent, and believe me, books of eras past were not afraid to tell you that you were a bad mother* to your face. Do you want to be known as the bad parent? Of course not.

The second problem is that there were perceived health consequences for your child if they slept poorly, and they were (or at least sounded) quite dire. Depending on what you read, some ailments of sleep-deprived children included "eyes that are red and gummy," "obtuseness of mind," "debased [demeanor]," "a sloven," "dull, languid, stupid." Poor sleep frayed the nerves and was an invitation for mental illness, disease, and death, not to mention fussiness.

The bottom line was that poor sleep, whatever the definition, was to be avoided like consumption, brain dropsy, and winter fever. Thinking about it as a parent, it makes sense. What is more troubling than a child who is not sleeping when she is supposed to? It not only feels medically problematic, but it's also a huge inconvenience for a busy caregiver. In that sense, serving the baby up with some medical-grade malt liquor seems almost rational.

That was then. Fast-forward a few decades, and things got serious when it came to knocking kids out. Nembutal (pentobarbital) was a commonly used sedative for anxious children dating back to the 1930s and probably helped replace the use of opium derivatives for sedation. Over time, these drugs, largely due to safety issues (they were likely responsible for the death of Marilyn Monroe), fell out of favor as sleep aids.†

With a renewed focus on the safety of children, the next generation of

* Not to be confused with being a bad mutha like Mike Tyson or Tim Gunn.

† Drugs have a way of repurposing themselves for other uses, and pentobarbital is no exception. It is often used in executions today.

pediatricians seemed to shy away from the heavy-duty barbiturates and benzodiazepines (think: Valium), and move toward the much safer antihistamine family of drugs. Over time, these drugs exploded in over-the-counter preparations. Got a drug? Add some antihistamine to it, throw a PM on the bottle, and suddenly you have a new drug to market and to occupy more space for your brand name on a drugstore shelf.

While antihistamine drugs are still in use, these days it is all about melatonin, the naturally occurring chemical in our brain that links darkness to sleep. Suddenly it's everywhere—added to other pediatric medications, put in sports drinks, injected into cute gummy bears and given out like candy. One point of concern regarding melatonin—when a child is given melatonin artificially, it potentially sends a disruptive message to his brain to produce less natural melatonin because he is getting it via another source. To date, no studies have demonstrated or disproven this theory, and adult studies have not been robust.

Is any of this truly helpful? Hard to say. Studies vary, and one reason they vary is because the amount of melatonin in the pill you are giving your adolescent varies wildly from one brand to the next (with many having no melatonin in them at all). Beyond that, even within the same brand of melatonin, the pill-to-pill amount can vary by over 400 percent! The main reason I am against sleeping pills of all shapes and sizes is that 99 percent of the time they are given, recommended, or prescribed, there is no medically valid reason for doing so and little to no science to support the use of the drug. One of my favorite Secret Laws of Sleep is: "I've never met a sleeping pill that doesn't lie."*

"My child can't sleep."
"Oh my! Here, try some melatonin gummies."

Imagine reacting this way to any other medical complaint.

---

* I'll reveal some more of my Secret Laws of Sleep as we go along. They aren't really secret laws. They are just expressions I commonly use with my sleep patients.

"My child is developing a rash."

"Oh my! Here, try this linen jumpsuit."

Much better. No more unsightly and distressing rash. He looks great now.

The problem is, was anything truly solved, or did we just cover it up? If you only respond to a single symptom without digging deeper and getting context, prescribing pills is no better than putting a bandage on a broken bone. Pills often do far worse than cover up a problem. They let conditions fester and grow. Bottom line—kids should not be on sleeping pills without a damn good medically justified reason, and in my entire career, I have only heard a handful of reasons that even approached that criteria.

Why not? I mean, what's the harm?* Putting aside addictiveness, drug interactions, and side effects, there is a huge harm that is rarely talked about. Giving a child a sleeping pill is tantamount to saying, "Something is wrong with your ability to sleep, so I am giving you ___ to fix it" (fill in whatever medication, supplement, or gummy you like). This statement is a lie. No child needs a drug to fall asleep. Sleep is inevitable. By condoning that pill, I am further undermining this kid's ability to develop a positive sleep identity and likely increasing the chances that he will be in somebody's waiting room one day arguing that he "absolutely needs" some outrageous drug combination to fall asleep. That patient is a near-daily occurrence in my clinic.†

And what's the reason this adult patient is asking for these pills? "It's not because I want the pills, Doc. I hate being on them, but I need them to function." Parents are the same way. They want their kids to get good

* It's funny to me how few parents question the side effect of sleeping pills prescribed to their child, but their anti-seizure medications or vaccines are often worried over to the point of refusal.

† This is why the presence of adults in my clinic makes me a better kid-sleep doctor— I am reminded of the long-term consequences of poor early sleep education and therapy on a daily basis.

grades, have awesome trumpet recitals, crush their age group competitors in the swim meet this week, and get into the university of their dreams. They want their kids to function optimally.

Unfortunately, there is no research linking sleeping aids of any kind (even CBD!) to improved functioning. Go ahead. Ask that clinician giving your kid a medication for sleep, "Is this an approved drug specifically for sleep in children?" and (here's the kicker), "Can you direct me to some articles that demonstrate how this drug you are recommending for my child has been shown to improve her sleep at night and her functioning during the day?" If they actually have an answer, can you send me that paper? I have an empty file labeled "Studies on Sleeping Pills that Improve the Sleep, Health, and Performance of Children." I would love to have something to put in there. Until that time, in most situations, we can do better than a drug.

 "I don't think I can do what you are asking me to do."

Jackson's mother took in what I told her about Jackson's age and total sleep need. We talked about the amount she expected him to sleep at night and the schedule she wanted him to be on. She discussed the three-hour-long naps she wanted him to take, in concert with her one-year-old's sleep. Mainly we talked about consistency.

"But there is no way I can get what I need to get done if I'm always waking him up to keep on a schedule. What about melatonin? That's what my sister uses for her kids."

More discussion follows. I offer that if she feels her life is better with Jackson having no schedule for his sleep, she is not obligated by any law to adopt my plan. She just needed to understand that with an irregular and unpredictable schedule will come an irregular and unpredictable child. Just like the one in front of us.

Eventually, she agreed. I almost lost her when, fairly quickly, it became apparent that Jackson was going to rest twice during the day and no more. She did not like this development and was highly irritated when instead of a melatonin lollipop, I gave her some talk about rest time, not sleep time.

But she hung in there, and she listened with an open mind. And Jackson eventually slept, as did his sister, with whom the same principles were applied with smashing results.

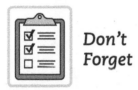 **Don't Forget**

1. As soon as you begin to talk to your baby, even if he has not been born yet, tell him what an awesome sleeper he is. It's never too early to think about his sleep identity.

2. Don't sleep with your child in your bed. Love her in other ways.

3. Naps are good, but they should be scheduled and not take away from sleep at night.

4. A child doesn't need a pill to sleep. Every parent has the right to understand exactly why a medication is being given to their child. Why is your doctor giving your child a sleep aid?

Pediatric Insomnia

Understanding What It Means When Your Child Says He "Can't Sleep"

 Jasmine is a spirited four-year-old girl who has struggled with her sleep all her young life. During our appointment, Mom, a nurse, tells the story as Jasmine moves around my exam room excitedly. Jasmine climbs onto her mother's lap. She looks at a book. She drops the book. She is doing what can only be described as a dumpster dive into her mother's purse. She victoriously emerges with a cell phone and a coupon for Dick's Sporting Goods. As she effortlessly logs into the phone, she announces that she needs, "a football, soccer ball, and basketball from Dick's." She says this while adding details and her opinions to what her mother is claiming about her sleep.

"We put Jasmine to bed at eight p.m., and it is not uncommon for her to still be up at midnight. Sometimes she's out of bed at four a.m., ready to go. The girl does not sleep."

At one point, her mother said something about falling asleep in a car.

"No, I don't. I never sleep, and you said if I don't start, bad things will happen and you will take my toys away."

"Sweetheart, I didn't say that."

I note that Jasmine had a sleep study six months earlier, and I ask what it showed.

"Nothing. They never said anything about it. She barely slept!"

Fortunately, Jasmine's pediatrician sent over some notes and a copy of the sleep study in question. Among the highlights were:

JASMINE SLEEP STUDY

Lights-out time: 11:10 p.m.
Time asleep: 11:42 p.m.
Sleep efficiency: 98.07 percent
Total sleep time: 7 hours 10 minutes
Tech notes: Mother snores loudly

Sleep efficiency: 98.07 percent. In other words, after Jasmine fell asleep, she slept 98 percent of the time until she awakened for good. Put another way, Jasmine was out cold.

~ ~ ~

While snoring and sleep apnea might be the most common complaint in my adult clinic population, insomnia is—without question—the most common complaint of the pediatric clinic. Nothing is more distressing to a child (and their caregivers) than not being able to sleep. Think about everything that is riding on her ability to sleep: her health, her grades, her college, her future! This is heavy stuff, and it all hinges on shutting that racing mind off when the lights go out. We've all been there . . . waiting . . . frustrated . . . angry . . . scared.

All nights mercifully come to an end—and this end is routinely a debriefing of the night over breakfast. Often a child will complain of "not sleeping," or maybe he will say that he never slept at all. This is not an uncommon occurrence. It is estimated that approximately 50 percent of kids will have trouble sleeping at some point. Frankly, I'm surprised the number is that low. Can you imagine a kid graduating college without a sleepless night over a test gone poorly or a relationship that crashed and burned?

Given the high frequency of sleep difficulties that we see in children of all ages, and the relative importance we place on sleep as the secret ingredient to everything related to health, success, and happiness, it is easy to see why the sleep aids mentioned in the previous chapter are so ubiquitous: kids desperately want to sleep, parents are terrified of the notion of their kids not sleeping, and doctors, when they become involved, feel like they are obligated to do something to remedy the situation. But what exactly is the situation? Can a child really "not sleep" at night?

Let's unpack Jasmine's story. Just to be clear, stories like Jasmine's are very common. Names and numbers might vary a little from one case to the next, but they are remarkably consistent.

The first question I ask any parent when they walk through the door is, "What seems to be the problem with your child's sleep?" or simply, "What can I do for you?" Jasmine has been brought to my clinic because she cannot sleep. Jasmine's mother said then (and several other times during the interview) that Jasmine does not sleep. She even remarked about her not sleeping during the sleep study. "Can't sleep" is a common problem with kids of all ages. When they're babies, it seems like something we simply need to accept, or that it is something they will grow out of. As kids mature, the condition often slowly morphs from something that is unfortunate yet expected, to something that is much more malignant and scary.

 Richardson wrote extensively about sleep need in her vintage musings. The idea of a child not sleeping was, in her mind, an absolute absurdity. She writes, "It is nonsense to say that a young child does not want to sleep—nature cries out for sleep."

She goes on to draw a parallel between a child's desire for sleep and their need for food: "Take it for granted that he was sent into the world with sound nerves and a normal appetite for sleep as well as food."

The take-home message is simple, though it is a double negative: Your child is *not* capable of *not* sleeping.*

What Is Pediatric Insomnia?

For many parents, the term "insomnia" refers to a child who "can't sleep" or perhaps "won't sleep." So is it possible for a child to truly stop sleeping? No. Sleep is a scientific certainty. If that is true, then what is happening here? Simply put, Jasmine is sleeping, but she is not sleeping well. This a very important distinction. However, "well" is a little ill-defined, so let's dig a bit deeper and refine our definition of insomnia.

Jasmine is not sleeping immediately when she is put to bed. Stated another way, her sleep is unpredictable, both to herself and her parents. This is a problem. For young children, there is a real performance anxiety that can develop. They are being asked to fall asleep at a certain time, but they are struggling to do so. That sense of failure creates frustration. As children mature, this failure gets attached to tangible measures of health and productivity compromise.† It can be equally problematic for parents. Mom has a thing she needs to get done, and knowing that Jasmine will be asleep at certain times (either at night or during daytime naps) is a real positive. It allows her parents to plan out their activities, work, chores, etc. Not knowing when or if Jasmine is going to rest on any given day not only makes planning impossible but also creates a tremendous lack of productivity. This lack of productivity creates frustration that eventually is fed back to the child struggling to rest.

I see parents on a regular basis who, when asked how I can help them, reply, "Please help me get my child to sleep." Parents absolutely need to understand that their child *not sleeping* is not the issue. Your child *not sleeping when you want her to* is the real issue. In other words, you are miserable now because it is your daughter's bedtime, but she is not getting that message and falling asleep on cue. The problem is not that she won't sleep, it is that she won't sleep *now*.

* Chris's Secret Law of Sleep #2: Your kid couldn't "not sleep" even if he tried.

† Fatalistic mirroring returns.

Please think about this concept carefully, because it gets at the core of what we commonly refer to as insomnia.* If you believe my statement that your child, and every child, sleeps, what are we really talking about here? We are talking about timing. We want our child to sleep, more or less, when it works for us. When they do not, it is very easy to lazily declare to other parents at a preschool pickup that "My child can't sleep." Nobody will really be that shocked. You might get a supportive nod from some folks, but it is doubtful someone would shake their head as they ran up to you and said, "No way . . . all kids sleep. What you are saying is impossible." It is the way we talk about sleep.

In addition to Jasmine's sleep being unpredictable, it is also inefficient. The total time she spends in bed is far more than the total time she sleeps. In other words, there is a lot of wasted time spent staring at the glow-in-the-dark star stickers on her ceiling.

So when a parent (or an adult for that matter) tells you that their kid is a terrible sleeper, or can't sleep, what they are really saying is that their child has unpredictable sleep and/or inefficient sleep. With that in mind, let's take a quick peek at Jasmine's "indeterminate" sleep study results.

Was her sleep unpredictable? She was put into bed at 11:10 p.m. and fell asleep at 11:42 p.m. This is not particularly distressing to a sleep specialist, but the fact that it takes over half an hour for her to fall asleep at 11:10 p.m. could be quite distressing to a parent, especially if the thirty minutes are filled with "I need more water," or "Can we look under the bed and in the closet to make sure there is nobody in there?" For the sake of argument, let's say that yes, Jasmine's sleep shows signs of being unpredictable.

Was her sleep inefficient? Once she fell asleep, she slept 98 percent of the time she had available to her to sleep. From that perspective, no, her sleep was extremely efficient. If we look at the entire night, however, she

---

* Interestingly, parents never seem to use the term "insomnia" with little ones. Monikers like "bad sleeper" are much more common. It seems like the term "insomnia" usually goes along with getting one's learner's permit.

was awake for over half an hour before she fell asleep. By that metric, no, she was not particularly efficient: she wasted a lot of time up front.*

So if Mom was literally in the room with Jasmine during the sleep study (parents/guardians always stay with kids during sleep studies), why did she tell me that Jasmine didn't sleep? Why does Jasmine think she's not sleeping, for that matter? Are they making everything up?

Absolutely not. To understand what is happening here, it is very important to understand Chris's Secret Law of Sleep #3:

Perception of sleep and reality of sleep are two completely different things.

Sleep Perception

Ever take a ride in an amusement park go-kart—you know, the ones you take your family to ride in at the beach? When it is all over, your youngest will inevitably complain that her kart was slower than the karts the rest of the family drove, and that's why she always lost when you raced. Relative speed and competitive fairness aside, think about how it feels to drive that kart around the figure-eight course. You feel like you are going one hundred miles an hour, way faster than you feel driving your big SUV down the highway.

Consider that the kart you were racing at the beach was only going about thirty-five miles an hour, tops, while your speed in the SUV was approaching seventy. How could the feeling be so off? Why is the perception of speed in the go-kart so much greater than in the SUV?

Sleep works in a similar way. When an individual is stressed, uncomfortable, or in unfamiliar surroundings, the brain can sometimes fail to recognize lighter stages of sleep as being sleep. In some cases, the results are extreme, with individuals failing to recognize any sleep for months or even years. Now put yourself into the position of the parent of a child

---

* It is worth noting that the way sleep efficiency (SE) is calculated is taking total sleep time (TST) and dividing it by the total time spanned from sleep onset to the final awakening. Therefore, an individual could take two hours to fall asleep but still have a high sleep efficiency.

who complains of getting no sleep on a nightly basis. This can be very stressful.

One final piece of analysis—if we look back at Jasmine's sleep study, it mentioned that Mom, who accompanied Jasmine, snored very loudly. We see this frequently in sleep labs. The daughter comes in to be evaluated, but at the end of the night, the sleep technician is far more concerned about the accompanying parent than the kid in question. In this example, we ended up diagnosing Jasmine's mother with sleep apnea. Sleep apnea, as will be discussed later, can absolutely decimate someone's sleep quality. It is not too hard to imagine, with Mom's sleep quality already in serious jeopardy, how that might influence her own sleep and her own view and interpretation of her daughter's sleep issues.

So to summarize, we have a mother complaining that her child cannot sleep, yet (1) we know that's scientifically impossible, and (2) we have a sleep study showing that she does in fact sleep, and quite efficiently to boot. This is a touchy place to be in as a clinician. As a sleep doctor, I need to make sure the parents are heard, but at the same time, I need to help them understand that while there is an issue afoot, it is not the issue they think it is.

Diagnosing Pediatric Sleep-Onset Insomnia

Much is written about the diagnostic criteria for insomnia in children and teens. I honestly think the majority of it is nonsense. Language about the condition "lasting three months or more" or "affects an individual more than three nights/week" is really missing the point. To me, insomnia is like migraines. If you can deal with a bunch of migraines every week, that's your call. If one migraine a month is too much to bear, then let's figure out a treatment that works for you.

Simply put—your child has insomnia when his sleep is not satisfactory to either him or you. When that time comes, it is time to seek help. If you think your child is struggling with insomnia, then he's struggling with insomnia. End of story.

Treating Pediatric Insomnia

When parents seek treatment for their children who "can't sleep," most primary care docs will handle this situation in one of two ways: pill or punt.

With pills, the doctor will simply give the child something to take that will make the child sleepy and want to sleep. Melatonin seems to be in vogue right now, but there are many others that do the trick: Benadryl, clonidine, Ambien, clonazepam . . . and so on! The goal here is to sedate the child so that you stop calling the pediatrician, and the pediatrician can get on with her overscheduled day. There's no talk about insomnia definitions, and often no real plan except for a follow-up in three to six months. Most important, there's no real diagnosis. Just the symptom of sleeplessness being treated with sedatives.*

With the punt option, the clinician does not engage, either because he does not want to, doesn't have time to do so (treating sleep disturbances takes time), or doesn't know how. If he doesn't know how or does not have the time, that's completely understandable. Keep in mind that a 2016 study (conducted by pediatrician and professor Dirk Bock) found that only 20 percent of pediatricians have ever gotten any training regarding the prescribing of sleeping pills in children, yet 66 percent routinely prescribe them.† They don't know what they are doing. You do not want me to deliver your baby or manage your ventilator—that is not my wheelhouse—I have no real training in those areas of medicine. So if those issues arise, I'm going to send you to someone who has that training—I'll punt to you.

If the reason, however, is because the clinician does not want to treat the problem, in my mind, that's unacceptable. So hopefully punting simply

---

* Secret Law of Sleep #4: Sleep and sedation are not the same thing.

† It reminds me of that study a pilot conducted that concluded only 20 percent of pilots flying the Airbus A330 transatlantic commercial passenger airplane had ever gotten any training on the aircraft. This study is not real. Unfortunately for children, the pediatric study about sleeping pill training is real.

means he's sending you to me or someone else who specializes in the sleep needs of kids.

Chances are that either way, your child will eventually visit a sleep specialist, either because of the immediate punt or the doctor's pills will eventually fail and the kid will end up needing a referral.* Awesome, because that's what we're here for! So what do we do about this?

First things first, I have to make sure that all parents and children involved understand the Golden Rule of Sleep: Everybody sleeps.† Put another way, while your sleep may be problematic, the problem we are not dealing with is someone who can't sleep. This is important. Hearing this fact from a sleep doctor usually provides a sense of comfort to a child or parent. Sometimes it does not. Occasionally, it is met with anger, hostility, and total disbelief. I can understand that. From the parent's perspective, they feel like they are dealing with a child who simply cannot shut their mind off. It has been hard for them—missed school, diminished activities, doctors and specialist visits, and sometimes a very bleak outlook on the future. To walk into an office and be told that all this stress over your child's inability to sleep has been misplaced because they do in fact sleep can be irritating!

What is the path forward? There are concrete, practical, and effective ways to begin to improve the situation.

Whether you have children who have sleep problems, it is imperative that you instill within them a sense of confidence when it comes to sleep. Avoid phrases like:

"If we don't get you back to sleep you're liable to catch a cold or coronavirus." (Anxiety card)
"Buster, you better march your ass right back up those stairs and get to sleep. If I find you awake in the next ten minutes when I

---

* In keeping with the football analogy, I suppose that is the equivalent of a turnover on downs: you went for it with the pills, but came up short.

† Or stated as Secret Law of Sleep #5: Sleep always wins.

check on you, you're grounded for a week—no phone." (Anger
card)

"Listen up, we've got a situation! A fourteen-year-old with an algebra test tomorrow is dying upstairs, and we are his only chance.
Talk to me, people, give me some ideas. I'm sure we have something around here that can help. Here's some Benadryl liquid
that expired a few years ago, but it smells okay. How about warm
milk? What about that smelly stuff you rub on a kid's chest, does
that make any sense?" (Apollo 13–working-the-situation card)

These tactics are not helpful, and they can be damaging not only in
the short term but also over much longer periods of time as they may
start creating anxieties related to sleep. While it may be difficult, encouraging words like, "It is okay that you are having trouble falling asleep
tonight, but don't worry, it always comes. Why don't you look at your
book?" is a much better way to address a difficult night.

One night, my sixteen-year-old son came downstairs while I was
watching *The Voice*, and exasperatedly told me he simply could not sleep.
In this situation, I went with none of the aforementioned methods. I
calmly said, without even taking my eyes off the battle rounds, "Doesn't
your English teacher require you to write an essay of your choice every
two weeks?"

"Uh, yeah," he said questioningly.

"Since it is already midnight, why don't you read some comic books
and just stay up the rest of the night. You could write your essay about
what it is like to stay up all night on a school night. That would be cool."

If I may paint a verbal picture of my son's face, it can only be described
as a look of utter confusion followed by the realization that his father
might be the worst goddamn sleep doctor in the world. There was a hint
of disappointment when I did not procure him some supersecret sleeping pills.

"Uh, okay."

"I love you. Good luck. Come back down if you need anything else."

He walked away. He was soundly asleep twenty minutes later when I
was preparing for bed.

What just happened? Many things, actually. By not playing the anxiety card, I removed any interpretation that what was going on was scary, dangerous, or really all that unusual. I've never met a kid who came out of his room to tell his parents that he sneezed. We accept sneezing as a normal thing even if it is an unusual occurrence. I wanted my son to think of this situation as normal as well.

By not playing the anger card, I took away the performance anxiety. It is good that we do this for children in general.

Finally, by not playing the Apollo 13 card, I'm teaching my son that you don't have to do something; there is no solution necessary because there really is no problem here. I tell patients all the time that to never have a sleeping problem is kind of weird. Having one from time to time is much more commonplace.

This is all to say that we are addressing this issue by removing fear from the equation. It is essential that regardless of our own beliefs, we do not associate (even accidentally) the idea of having difficulty sleeping with the feeling of fear. By doing so, you are not only providing a woefully inadequate solution to the situation at hand, but you are kindly providing some sleep doctor of the future a new patient who will describe herself as "someone who has always been a bad sleeper."

As the difficult night passes, we must work hard to seek the positives and project the title of super sleeper onto our children, even if the moniker doesn't fit every night. To help a child form a positive sleep identity, we must always search for opportunities to remind our kids how good their sleep is and how well they do it. On the nights they don't crush it, largely ignore it.

The tone has been set. Now what? Easy. Now it is time to figure out how much sleep your child needs. For many kids who struggle to sleep, there is a simple mismatch between how much sleep a child needs and the opportunity for sleep they are given. Let me explain.

When you put a child into bed at 9:00 p.m., they are going to sleep a specific amount that is not endless. At some point, they will wake up and be done sleeping. This is not different from eating or drinking. At some point, we finish. Sleep is the same way.

Since insomnia refers to a child not sleeping when or how long they

National Sleep Foundation Recommended Hours of Sleep		
Age	Recommended	May Be Appropriate
Newborn (0–3 months)	14–17 hours	11–19 hours
Infant (4–11 months)	12–15 hours	10–18 hours
Toddler (1–2 years)	11–14 hours	9–16 hours
Preschool (3–5 years)	10–13 hours	8–14 hours
School Age (6–13 years)	9–11 hours	7–11 hours
Teen (14–17 years)	8–10 hours	7–11 hours
Young Adult (18–25 years)	7–9 hours	6–11 hours

Hirshkowitz, M., Whiton, K., Albert, S. M., Alessi, C., Bruni, O., DonCarlos, L., Hazen, N., Herman, J., Katz, E. S., Kheirandish-Gozal, L., Neubauer, D. N., O'Donnell, A. E., Ohayon, M., Peever, J., Rawding, R., Sachdeva, R. C., Setters, B., Vitiello, M. V., Ware, J. C., & Adams Hillard, P. J. (2015). National Sleep Foundation's sleep time duration recommendations: methodology and results summary. *Sleep health*, *1*(1), 40–43.

are "supposed to," the sleep amount we set for that child is important and may need to change. Remember this graph from page 13? This is such a powerful diagram. First, it illustrates the dramatic differences in sleep need from one child to the next. Second, it does a great job conveying the dramatic decrease of sleep need seen over the maturation of a child.

Let's revisit Jasmine. Jasmine is four years old. What clues do we have about the amount of sleep Jasmine needs? To start, it is probably safe to assume that Jasmine is not a fourteen-hour sleeper.* If she was, this appointment would never have happened. It's safe to assume that Jasmine's on the lower end of sleep need.

We also have the results of the sleep study. Granted, this represents one unusual night of wires, cameras, glue, and some mildly annoying flickering lights. Accepting the out-of-the-ordinary nature of the circumstances, it is safe to assume that the strangeness of the night hindered sleep rather than facilitated sleep, right? Keep in mind too that sleep studies are extra stressful for children. You can tell a kid a million times that the process will be painless, that Mommy or Daddy will be with them all night, and that there will be absolutely no shots or needles of any kind involved. Despite this, in the backs of their minds, each and every child

---

* Often referred to as a "good sleeper," "great sleeper," or "dream child."

thinks the whole affair is just a ploy to ruthlessly get them into the room, strap them to a bed, and for Mommy to disappear while I fill a foot-long rusty syringe with medicine to be injected into their arm.

Despite this perceived diabolical plot, Jasmine slept seven hours and ten minutes.

Another truth about sleep studies is that most parents have to wake the kids up relatively early to get them unhooked and processed so that the tech can leave (she's been there since probably 5:00 or 6:00 p.m. the day before . . . well before Jasmine arrived). With this in mind, there is a great chance that had the tech not had to go home, Jasmine could have slept even longer!

So where are we at? We have a girl whose parents claim is not able to sleep, though she does in fact sleep, probably some amount over seven hours but probably far less than fourteen. Let's think a moment about that 98.07 percent sleep efficiency. What that tells me is that Jasmine has a high drive to sleep once she falls asleep. It is like examining the dinner plates of two children: let's call them Marcus and Tamara. In addition to half his chicken, Marcus leaves most of his peas on his plate, and a few potatoes. Conversely, Tamara's plate is literally licked clean. If they both started with the same amount of food, what do you imagine these plates says about their relative appetites? When we see high sleep efficiencies, we generally suspect a high sleep drive. So maybe this is a vote for Jasmine needing a bit more than seven hours. I'm going to take a stab and say her amount is eight—the bottom of the sleep amount indicated on the chart. In other words, I think Jasmine needs less than the average amount of sleep for a child her age.

Guess what? We have a name for people like this. At the risk of sounding scholarly and overtechnical, the name is *short sleepers*. I'm making an assumption that Jasmine is a short sleeper and simply does not need the same amount of sleep as other four-year-olds in her preschool. Why do I think this?

1. Jasmine is not able to sleep through the night. Her sleep is inefficient, so despite being given time from 8:00 p.m. to 6:00 a.m. to

sleep, she simply does not utilize that entire ten hours. If we frame that in terms of:

a. Sleep opportunity = ten hours

b. Sleep need = eight hours (my guess)

We can see how things might be unpleasant. If we think about Jasmine only needing eight hours of sleep, this schedule has set her up to fail from the start.

2. If you look at the results of the sleep study, it took Jasmine a while to fall asleep. That is absolutely to be expected given the stress-inducing nature of a sleep study in a four year-old.* However, she did fall asleep a little before midnight and slept really well.† That later bedtime at the sleep center is probably more in line with the time Jasmine should actually be going to bed. This is part of the reason why kids often surprise their parents and sleep well during a sleep study.

3. Mom is a nurse. This is not typically a career full of long sleepers! Nursing school tends to weed them out quickly. I remember how hard college was for my friends in the nursing school. Tons of classes, and on top of those, they were working long hours in the

---

* This is why it is imperative that a sleep lab have outstanding sleep techs who will put the minds of kids (and parents) at ease prior to the study. That process starts with your sleep clinician as well. She should have kids and parents relaxed and comfortable with the sleep study before the first wire is glued on. If you are not getting that kind of support and education, find a different sleep doc—that stress will absolutely affect the quality of your kid's sleep study.

† It's amazing how many parents are absolutely befuddled that their kid who can't sleep sleeps remarkably well at the sleep center with wires glued to their scalp.

hospital.* To survive and graduate, you needed to be able to function at a high level on relatively small amounts of sleep. I suspect other professions like law and the military tend to attract short sleepers. If Mom is in fact a short sleeper, this tendency is a genetic trait—and guess which four-year-old may have inherited it?

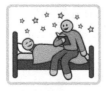 It is time to figure out how much sleep your child needs. Forget what the daytime television doctor or the sleep coach told you. Take a look at the National Sleep Foundation's chart and find your kid's age. Your kid's sleep amount is going to be somewhere in that range.

As far as finding the right number, there are a few ways to do it:

1. You can take a guess. Maybe aim for something that has them in bed an hour or two less than what they are currently getting as a jumping-off point. I would not recommend this method.

2. Change nothing about what you are doing with your child, and simply grab a notebook and a pencil, and become an amateur sleep scientist, meticulously recording every minute of your child's sleep over the next two to four weeks. When I say every minute, I mean *every minute*:

SUNDAY

Time in bed: 9:00 p.m.
Fell asleep 10:40 p.m.
Woke up 2:20 a.m. and tried to get into bed with us
Back to sleep at 4:00 a.m.
Woke up briefly at 5:00 a.m.
Out of bed at 6:30 a.m.

---

* I never remember meeting nursing students at parties. I think they were way too busy to stand around with a red Solo cup.

Nap from 8:00–10:00 a.m.
Fell asleep in the car to grocery store, 15 minutes
Fell asleep going home, left in the running car with me, 1 hour
No afternoon nap

Once you have a few weeks of this journal, you can start to construct an average sleep time for your child per twenty-four hours. Let's take this example and break it down:

Slept 10:40–2:20	3 hours 40 minutes
Slept 4:00–6:30	2 hours 30 minutes. We can subtract a little since there was a brief awakening: 2 hours 15 minutes
Slept 8:00–10:00	2 hours
Slept 15 minutes	15 minutes
Slept 1 hour in car	1 hour
Total	9 hours 10 minutes

That's one night. It may be more or less than the representative average that you will calculate once you have determined the daily averages for your child over a few weeks. For this child, the average seems to be about nine hours.

QUICK CHECK

Is your child sleeping? Yes (Don't forget this).
Is your child's average within the range on the NSF chart on page 13? Yes.

Note: If you have read what I have written so far, and you remain in the camp of "no way my three-year-old sleeps nine hours," or have calculated a sleep time average lower than the lowest number in the range (less than eleven hours for a newborn for example), choose the lowest number in your child's sleep range. That will be his number. In other words, if your calculation yields nine hours for your newborn's average sleep time, use eleven, the lowest in the reported range.

3. Purchase some kind of sleep monitor. Later in the book, we dive into the plastic sleep saviors on everyone's wrist. For now, let's keep it simple. Buy the device, charge it, download the free app, and strap it on your kid's nondominant wrist. If you are dealing with a baby, there are passive monitors that can sit on a table next to your child and record sleep. Now forget about it for a few weeks. When the few weeks are up, take a look at the results. Add up the total amount of sleep registered over the last three weeks. That's twenty-one data points:

9 hours 17 minutes	8 hours 43 minutes	6 hours 38 minutes
8 hours 45 minutes	7 hours 03 minutes	8 hours 30 minutes
9 hours 16 minutes	5 hours 50 minutes	9 hours 01 minute
9 hours 09 minutes	10 hours 03 minutes	8 hours 27 minutes
9 hours 22 minutes	9 hours 45 minutes	9 hours 40 minutes
10 hours 11 minutes	9 hours 52 minutes	10 hours 16 minutes
9 hours 05 minutes	9 hours 43 minutes	10 hours 42 minutes

Add them up and divide by 21. Careful that you handle the hours and minutes properly. I find it easiest to convert everything to minutes, but maybe your calculator or spreadsheet is better than mine.

11,358 minutes ÷ 21 days = 540.86 minutes/day.

540.86 minutes ÷ 60 minutes/hour = 9.01 hours/day.

There you have it. This little one is sleeping nine hours and thirty-six seconds every twenty-four hours. Congratulations, you now have your child's initial sleep duration target time.

A quick note—remember the selective memory individuals have with relation to their sleep? It is very common for a parent to tell me that their kid is sleeping five to six hours a night, and then get data like what I just listed. Are there nights where the child slept five to six hours? Yes, one, maybe two, if you count the night with six hours and thirty-eight minutes.*

* But really that rounds up to seven, doesn't it?

Make no mistake, these are rough nights, particularly if you are expecting your child to sleep ten to eleven hours. Does a five- to six-hour night represent the average we just calculated? No, it doesn't. Hopefully this suggests the power these kinds of sleep issues carry with them in terms of sleep perception and recognition, and the resultant anxiety they can create.

Establishing this time is a big step for figuring out a healthy sleep schedule for your young child, teenager, or college student. It will give you and your child something to shoot for. More important, it will give you a starting point as you enter into negotiations with your child's brain. Think of her brain as a really demanding agent who happens to be representing her in this sleep negotiation.

> **Your child's brain:** We want a midnight bedtime, a television in our room, and unlimited sleeping in and naps, even on school days.
>
> **You:** I can do some limited sleeping in on weekends only, no naps unless sick or you got home late from an away soccer game, and a 9:00 p.m. bedtime with a 7:00 a.m. wake time. The TV is never going to happen.
>
> **Your child's brain:** What about a 10:00 p.m. bedtime? My client can live with the sleeping in and nap terms. We do want access to a TV in our bedroom if we have a friend over.
>
> **You:** Draw up the contract.

Boom! You did it. You have established a concrete sleep time for your kid. Nine hours . . . from 10:00 p.m. until 7:00 a.m. That's the easy part—now you have to enforce it! And just like any contract, that's often the hard part.

 Jasmine was very excited to show off her new wrist-worn sleep tracker the next time I saw her.

"It is pink," she said matter-of-factly.

In fact, it was.

"How much sleep is she averaging lately?"

Usually around seven and a half to eight hours.*

"How has sleep been, everybody?"

Mom took over. "Sleep has been much better. We have decided on a ten p.m. bedtime with Jazz getting up at six a.m. She's been doing much better, and so have we."

"And my teacher says I'm soooooooooooooooo much better."

"Yes, she does." Her mother grinned. "It usually doesn't take Jazz long to fall asleep, never more than twenty to thirty minutes. We have worked hard to keep her from napping and sleeping in the car. We have been good about weekends too."

"Whose bed are you sleeping in now?" I asked Jasmine.

"I sleep in my bed because I don't like Mom's 'C-Pack.'"

After Jasmine's sleep study and Mom's resultant sleep apnea diagnosis, she is now the proud owner of a new CPAP (continuous positive airway pressure) device to treat her apnea. It is pink too.

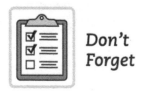 **Don't Forget**

1. Your child sleeps.

2. Your child's perception of his sleep (and your perception of his sleep) may differ significantly from the reality of his sleep.

3. Every parent seeks predictable and efficient sleepers.

4. It is essential to take the time to calculate how much sleep your child needs at her particular age.

* Seven and a half hours . . . just like in the sleep study.

4

Sleep Schedules

A Scheduled Child Makes a Happy Parent.

 Charlie is holding his family hostage. I could tell because during our meeting, his mother was doing that thing hostages do with their eyes that lets you know, *I'm talking to you casually, but it is all an act. There's a crazy person in the room with me, and I need you to call the police for help.*

Charlie was seven and effortlessly tearing his family apart.

"He won't go to sleep. He won't stay in his bed. He won't nap."

The list of grievances was robust.

It was interesting to watch Charlie as the prosecutor read the list of charges. Charlie was cold-blooded and completely in control. At one point he reached for his mother's cell phone and was told, "Not while we are talking to the doctor."

Without missing a beat, Charlie slid onto the floor and screamed. Within a minute he was smiling quietly as he played on the iPhone. "You get ten minutes."

No, actually he gets as much time as he wants, would be my guess.

Very quickly, the conversation becomes a long stream of sleep complaints Mom has about her precious son. As I begin to ask pretty routine questions like, "When does Charlie go to bed?" and "When does Charlie wake up?" it becomes clear that his mother is incapable of giving concrete answers to these questions. While there is incredible angst about Charlie's sleep, there is virtually no plan. No plan for bedtime, either what time that is or what it looks like. There is no plan for Charlie's near certain awakening during the night. How will that be handled? Wake times, napping, and weekend schedules are similarly unregulated.

Mom looks at me after being unable to answer most questions and says bluntly, "Listen, Doc. We're in survival mode here."

~ ~ ~

You have come a long way, and we are only in chapter 4! You already have a solid foundation of sleep science knowledge and understand many things you thought you knew about sleep, napping, and sleeping pills may have not been 100 percent accurate. You are thinking about your child's sleep and thoughtfully considering how much is the right amount for her. Whew. That's a lot.

With that specific sleep time you have determined, it is time to fashion a schedule around it. Let's think about this whole thing logically as we work out a plan, keeping in mind that while this seems to be a central focus of babies and their sleep, these principles apply equally—if not more—to sleepers of all ages.*

 Back in the day, sleep schedules were the norm.† Basically, if keeping your baby on a strict schedule did not cause your child to drop off to sleep *of his own sweet will,"* then there was something wrong with the baby, something wrong with Mom's breastmilk, or just something wrong with

---

* I say this because older children are a lot more motivated to make bad decisions and truly deprive themselves of sleep than babies. Remember that baby in Australia who was sneaking a phone into her crib and binge-watching *Love Island* episodes? Neither do I.

† Why is it always "back in the day," "in my day," "in days past," or "in the days of old"? Why don't nights ever get any love?

Mother in general. Dads were always fine back then. It was believed that newborns were going to sleep about twenty-two of twenty-four hours, and as baby matured, he would settle into "eight hours' sleep at night and a short nap in the middle of the afternoon."

What Is a Sleep Schedule and How Is It Constructed?

There are several steps involved with creating a sleep schedule that works for your child, and regardless of age, the steps are the same.

Establishing a Wake Time

The first and probably most important question to ask yourself when it comes to a child's sleep schedule is, "What time do I want their day to start?" One of the first questions I ask parents when I am learning about their child is very simple: "What time does he get up?" or perhaps, "What time do you get up, Dad, and start the day?" It is astonishing to watch parents often struggle to answer this question. Without a doubt, there have been answers that lasted fifteen minutes:

Well, if I have an early shift, I'm usually up around five a.m. and get Cameron up around five thirty a.m. I take him to my mother-in-law's house and drop him there. He will usually go back to sleep, but sometimes he just stays up and watches TV with his grandfather. On days I go in late we are usually up around seven or eight a.m. If I'm not working, I think Cameron has gotten up as late as eleven a.m., maybe noon, especially when he hasn't been sleeping so well.

This question needs a definitive answer, so please provide one in the space provided at your convenience. Take your time and really consider the answer.

Ideally, in order for my life and my child's life to function smoothly, it would be best if he/she/they wake(s) up at

_____.

_____Signed _____ Date _____Witness

Can you feel it? It is happening. A simple and logical approach to your child's sleep. You have thoughtfully calculated or recorded your child's average sleep time and begun to construct a schedule beginning with the wake time. Keep in mind, this time will be set in stone. It will not budge for anything or anybody. And remember that this wake time needs to suit the family's work and childcare needs rather than the child's personal preferences.

Determining a Bedtime

With that mission accomplished, let's turn our focus toward establishing and defining a bedtime.* Let's start with what the definition of bedtime should *not* be:

Bedtime (n): when your child goes to bed
    See also: "But I'm not tired," "Ten more minutes," and "Can I finish the rest of this episode? . . . It's almost over."

Instead, let's define a child's bedtime this way:

Bedtime (n): The earliest your child is allowed to go to bed.

Here's a good plan for younger school-aged kids (I'll discuss some strategies for other ages later in the chapter). When each of my kids turned nine or so, I sat them each down and had "the talk."† It went something like this:

[Child's name], you are practically an adult now, and there are some things Daddy wants you to know. First, you are my favorite child, but please never tell the others. It would hurt them deeply to know that. Second, I

---

* Be careful with this word. For some children, it is highly offensive and/or triggering.

† "The talk" in our house may differ from "the talk" in your home.

don't think you should have a bedtime anymore. You can stay up as late as you like. Now, Mommy and Daddy need you to be in your room without any phones, laptops, or screens of any sort by around seven to eight p.m. We also need you to stay in your room and not come out unless you smell smoke or there is someone in your room you don't recognize. Outside of that, feel free to read, draw, play with your action figures, or work on a puzzle as late as you like. Turn out the light whenever you are ready to sleep. It's up to you.

I can clearly remember the look on their faces when I was done. It was a look that combined elements of excitement, disbelief, wonder, and shock. "We get to stay up as late as we want?" For them, they felt like it was a dream come true. They could not wait to tell their friends.

I conveniently forgot to mention one small detail of the arrangement. Regardless of the night, they would be awakened at the same time every day. I would be pleasant when I woke them up; it was not meant to be a punishment. It was meant to be a message specifically targeted to their brains: *Be smart about the way you spend your time allotted for sleep, or pay the price.*

Once the rules were established, my wife and I completely backed off on the bedtime/lights-out thing. We made rules about when they had to be in their bedrooms, and where their electronics were plugged in for the night. But when they slept? . . . We pretended that we really didn't care too strongly one way or the other. This did not mean that we diminished the importance of sleep in our conversations with the kids. We just talked about it in very reassuring terms, that no matter the struggle, sleep generally works. Even when it seems like it is not, it is. The stock market takes big dips, but ask any broker the overall nature of the market: it is up . . . it works.

And it will work for your kids. From the last chapter, you have the sleep diary and/or the Fitbit data that you've acquired that gives an estimate of how much time in bed they need. That time should be reassuring as well as instructive. For this exercise, we can use nine hours. Assuming a 7:00 a.m. agreed-upon wake time that you signed off on earlier, we are going to work backward from there—nine hours. Voilà, 10:00 p.m. is the new bedtime!

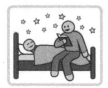 Now it is your turn to do some math and figure out when your child should be going to bed. It's up to you if you want to build in a little extra "downtime" in their room prior to their bedtime for reading, meditation, or next-day outfit selection.

a) MY CHILD'S WAKE TIME IS _____.

b) MY CHILD'S TOTAL SLEEP TIME AT NIGHT IS _____ HOURS.

c) MY CHILD'S BEDTIME IS _____.

Check your answers. If your child goes to bed at [c] and sleeps for [b] hours, are they waking up at [a]? If so, you did it!

So here is the complete list of sleep schedule rules:

1) No sleep or time in bed until bedtime (e.g., 10:00 p.m.). Even if your kid is exhausted and begging to sleep, don't allow it. It is your job to keep them up. You can be sly about it. "Want to play a game?" Or overt: "Remember the sleep doctor from the book says you can't sleep now."*

2) Make sure to get all the presleep activities (bath, pajama selection, dental care, etc.) out of the way in advance of bedtime. Leave no room for stalling.

3) At bedtime (e.g., 10:00 p.m.) your child asks (or you ask your child) the simple question: "Do I (you) feel sleepy?"

    a. If yes: go to the bedroom, get into bed, turn out the light.

---

* Go ahead and throw me under the bus! I don't mind being the bad guy!

    b. If no: go to the bedroom, climb onto bed, read *Dr. Seuss's Sleep Book.*

And if they stay up, everyone in the home needs to support the plan . . . encourage it. For an older child, suggest that this might be a great time to get caught up on that econ reading, or if they are younger, "Why don't you draw Mommy a picture of the cool train you saw today?" You should sound engaged and encouraging, but not nervous or upset they are not seeking sleep right now. The proper tone is matter-of-fact: Acknowledge "I see that you are not sleepy." Contextualize—"That's normal. It happens from time to time to us all." Then provide a plan: "This might be a good time to start writing your thank-you notes for the birthday gifts you received." For younger family members who cannot be trusted alone with pens or crayons, this is going to require some parental involvement. I know you really just want to sit down and watch *The Crown*, but trust me, this will all be worth it once your little one starts sleeping like a prince.

It is absolutely essential that your child should be made to feel that the fact they are still awake is normal, *because it is.* This is where sleep, for many kids, goes off the rails. While many books and "certified sleep coaches" tend to focus only on babies, this is a huge problem for high school– and college-aged students as well.* For older children an episode of poor sleep is looked upon as an urgent problem that needs to be fixed, rather than a natural occurrence that is going to happen from time to time. For sleep success, think about your child's sleep pattern as a mini Dow Jones Industrial Average. Forget the night-to-night variations (the Dow dropped one thousand points today! Panic!). Focus on the long-term trends (my daughter has slept quite well twenty-two of the last thirty days). Angst and stress do not work well on Wall Street, and they do not work well in your child's bedroom. In fact, it has been said that insomnia can only really exist in someone who is anxious about the whole affair. In other words, insomnia is not the inability to sleep but

---

* I mean, how many babies are worried that if they don't get enough sleep all of their friends will get good finance internships over the summer but they won't?

rather *the fear* of the inability to sleep. And with children, this fear is learned, usually from parents.

Implementing the Schedule

Establishing a bedtime and wake time is a great start in this sleep battle, but it means nothing if these times are not maintained. It is 7:00 a.m., your son is up in a brightly lit kitchen, food has been inserted into his tummy, and it is a mere four hours until his nap time. Uh-oh, as you were doing the dishes, he's fallen asleep in his chair at the table.

Think back to the statement we agreed upon. Your kid sleeps. Yippee! He's literally proving that I'm correct, right there in his high chair! Don't you feel better? Great, I'm glad you feel better. Now put the dish towel down and wake him up!

Remember our rule. No sleep outside the designated sleep periods. He had his chance to sleep last night. He chose not to utilize it. That was his choice. Now he gets to pay the consequence for that choice. The consequence is that he is going to feel sleepy and not be allowed to make that unpleasant feeling go away right now.

Careful, that smile on your face is fading . . . Don't let it. Wake him up with a hug and another handful of Honey Nut Cheerios! Yay! Being awake with Daddy is so much fun! With four hours to go until the next nap time, you are going to need to get really good at keeping your kid awake. Perhaps the hardest tactic to defend against is the car seat siesta. This is that thing kids do when you have to go to the store to get food and diapers and they exploit that situation to sleep in the car. Don't let that happen. I was ruthless in the car with my kids. I discovered that taking my daughter's socks off and playing with her feet would often make her cry when she was trying to sleep in the car. Cry away, sister . . . at least that pouting lets me know you are awake. When the sock removal didn't work, I would take a cold, damp washcloth and lay it across my kid's legs. They all universally hated that move. Not only was the temperature of the cloth wonderfully activating, the dampness coupled with their rudimentary abilities to grab items and remove them effectively made for a quick fix for a sleepy passenger. Remember, it is not about being mean. Make everything a fun game. If there are methods you can come up with that are more subtle that inspire wakefulness ("Let's see how many ambulances and police cars we can count on our trip to Whole Foods"), more power to you. I'll bet you can come up with better ideas than I have. If that idea is keeping them awake until their next nap, you win! If you fail, and your kid sleeps for ten minutes in the car, you may have a missed nap and a rage monster on your hands later that night.

Remember, enforcing the schedule is not age specific. Teens can be slippery. Are they really in their bedrooms doing homework on their bed? Better make sure.

Adjusting the Schedule

Now that the schedule is in place it's time to focus on assessing how the plan is working. A fourteen-day period is probably the best interval to use when adjusting any child's sleep schedule—long enough to see how things are truly going, but short enough to nimbly make changes when things are not working well. While this process can work for kids of all ages, keep in mind that younger children:

- typically need naps built into their schedule, and

- have sleep needs that are often rapidly changing, so what works well today may not be so perfect in six months. Be nimble!

If you happen to be one of those parents who sticks the landing on the first attempt, congratulations! You did it on the first try. You made an educated calculation as to what your child needs in terms of her sleep, and your math paid off. Your child is going to bed, and both you and she are satisfied with the way it is going in terms of how long it is taking her to fall asleep.*

* Notice that I did not assign this a time. In other words, we are not defining success in terms of your child falling asleep within fifteen minutes or something like that. I think this is a dangerous goal. Insomnia is not a concrete entity, but rather a feeling.

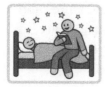 If your child is still struggling to fall asleep after fourteen days, some adjustments may need to be made. No problem! That is to be expected. Before we dive in, it is important to answer the following questions honestly.

YES/NO   My child is falling asleep prior to his bedtime.

YES/NO   My child is waking up after his wake time.

YES/NO   My child is napping/sleeping outside of his predetermined schedule.

If the answer is YES for any of these items, the process will not work. You absolutely must eliminate that extemporaneous sleeping. If, on the other hand, the answer is NO for all, it is time to make some adjustments.

For children who still nap, you have two options:

1. Evaluate nap times and eliminate fifteen to twenty minutes from a rest period.

2. Push your child's bedtime back fifteen to twenty minutes.

For children who do not nap, push their bedtime back thirty minutes.

As time passes, the schedule adjustments made to bedtime and/or nap times will act to consolidate his sleep. Do not think of it as taking away sleep from your child. Think of it as taking away empty time they were not using. It helps if you return to that idea of efficiency. We are trying to move the sleep opportunity time (the time they are in bed) as

---

If your child is awake for forty-five minutes before sleep comes, and is okay with that, you should be too. Remember part two of the insomnia definition! This definition of sleep success will serve your child well all his life.

close as possible to the actual amount of sleep that they need (total sleep time).

And if the opposite happens—your child falls asleep very quickly and is struggling now to stay awake at times during the day—your calculation of sleep need may have been too low. This happens occasionally, and it's okay.* If this is happening with your child, simply either add back in fifteen to twenty minutes of nap time or move the bedtime earlier by twenty to thirty minutes.

One final note—notice how we never adjust wake-up time. We want this to be a fixed time in your child's brain. This is essential for helping to regulate their circadian rhythm. By keeping this time set, we allow something very powerful to happen in your child's brain every single day she awakens. These dramatic state changes (light to dark, fasted to fed, etc.) have a powerful effect on sleep. How they can be manipulated to further strengthen your child's sleep and sleep schedule will be discussed later in the chapter.

How to Properly Handle Bedtime

There is much to do to prepare for the schedule's maiden voyage, and nothing's more important than formulating a bedtime ritual. While this is an important aspect of sleep in infants and toddlers, the underlying principles can be applied to kids of all ages.

Bedtime in children is a tricky thing. Despite being totally organized and prepared, there is a very good chance that you are going to be kept awake by a child who cries, calls out for you, asks for an endless number of items (glass of water, Band-Aid, pony), and/or shakes the crib endlessly. No worries. In anticipation of this potential obstacle, we just need to develop a philosophy for how these behaviors will be addressed.

There are surprising tricks and methods for getting a kid to fall asleep

* In adults, sleep doctors often aim for a total sleep time that intentionally under-sleeps patients just a little to jump-start their sleep drive and confidence so they can go to sleep without a pill.

everywhere. Entire books are based upon this topic. If you are a connois-
seur of these methods, here are a few you might be familiar with:

1. You can go the route of Richard Ferber and let your kid cry it
out.* Many people think this is cruel and unusual, akin to starving
your child if he refuses to eat his dinner. Because of the stress and
resultant cortisol release it induces, coupled with the known
negative effects of cortisol on a developing brain, there are theories
that this method potentially could cause brain damage. Despite
this, his book remains one of the top sellers.

2. The other popular method is from the book *On Becoming Baby
Wise*, which stresses schedules and making sure the baby puts
herself to sleep. This method works well, particularly if the child
can tell time and is handy with the schedule app on her iPhone.

3. There is also the "sleep whenever you want, wherever you want"
method, which touts that it is never okay to have expectations of
our children because it fosters a deep-rooted distrust of authority
and leads to teenagers who pierce their bodies and shoplift.

Here is the deal with these methods. They all have their merits when
applied with common sense in specific situations. Let's think about these
techniques and philosophies as we go through a typical night and imple-
mentation of a new schedule.

To begin the process, I want you to prep yourself. Repeat after me:

"Every child sleeps, and mine is no different."
[repeat]
"This too shall pass."
[repeat]
"This may take a while."
[repeat]

* Abbreviated CIO by bloggers everywhere. Other interesting acronyms are STTN
(sleep through the night) and DS (devil spawn).

"This problem will probably not be solved by the upcoming
   weekend."*
[repeat]
"My child does sleep."
[repeat]
"If this goes badly, I'm getting out of town for a weekend and
   getting Mom to do this. She's a tougher person than I am."
[repeat]

Enough affirmations. You are primed and ready to go. Your calculated bedtime arrives, and your kid looks pretty sleepy. Awesome. You put your child in bed, awake, after the requisite bedtime story. It is cheating if you nurse him to sleep and gently try to place your baby in the crib the same way Indiana Jones tried to steal that golden idol and replace it with a bag of sand.† Instead, gently pat him, sing to him, read to him, pray for him . . . whatever your ritual entails. I love a consistent bedtime ritual that does not change from night to night. When the ritual is done, kiss him good night and leave the room. I would advise you to demonstrate you are leaving by saying "bye-bye" or "good night." Don't sneak out.

The door closes. It is quiet! Ten minutes of silence have passed. OMG, you've done it! It worked! Dr. Winter is a bona fide genius.

And then . . .

"Uh."

What was that? Did you hear something? I think it was nothing . . . just the house settling, right?

"Wah."

That was the wind! you tell yourself, but dread and fear have crept into your soul. And suddenly, from the quiet bedroom erupts crying, or if

---

* But wow, don't you know *How to Get Your Kid to Sleep Perfectly by This Upcoming Weekend* would sell a lot of copies!

† At this point, you might prefer to take your chances with the huge rolling boulder rather than deal with your volatile kid in his Crib of Doom.

your child is a little older, talking, screaming, "I had a bad dream," "I can't sleep," "Can I sleep in your bed?" For high schoolers, you might hear them on their laptop or phone.

Take a deep breath.

Recite the mantra "Every child sleeps, and mine is no different."

Okay, your child is not sleeping *right now*. You get that. What are we going to do? Let's consider a child who is not sleeping, but she's not quite developed enough to get out of her crib/bed. Assuming that we have read the chapters in this book sequentially and worked through developing the perfect schedule for our kid, my vote is, to borrow a phrase from Sir Paul McCartney, "Let it be." I really dislike the term "cry it out." We should all replace that term with another more Beatles-esque term: "work it out."* "Cry it out" has such a cruel and heartless feel. When you let your child work it out, it means that you are giving them space to find their sleep rhythm in a supportive way. Does it mean that you rush to their aid at the first sound they make? No. Your child can cry. Your child is going to cry a lot in her lifetime. Does it really make sense that when you decide not to buy her a giant stuffed Minion at the store, and she cries, you are a bad parent and killing her brain cells? When she screams because she does not want to sit in her car seat, do you let her roam around the moving car unsecured because you fear buckling her in will lead to attention deficit disorder and lack of bonding? Of course not.

Expect your child to cry a little. It is okay. You know the difference between a gentle weep† and that hysterical hyperventilating scream with purple face and bulging forehead vein that happens when a kid is really hurt or upset. The working-it-out (WIO) method does not mean you let your child scream hysterically for hours. It doesn't. It does mean that there are periods you let your child cry, coupled with periods of support. Trust your instincts. You are going to know when to intervene.

At this point, you need to pick a time interval that you will wait before

---

* I also like "twist and shout," and it too seems appropriate here.

† More Beatles references. Maybe this book should be *The Sleep Solution: Golden Slumbers for Your Tot.*

going back into the room to console your child. There is nothing wrong with starting with five minutes, or even one minute. Whatever time you choose, you are not allowed to open that door prior to that time if possible. Use the time to find your inner happy place, because that is the image you very much need to project to the screaming child in the bedroom. My wife and I would sit outside our children's doors and just wait to see if they would work it out.

If not, after a designated time period, enter the room and console your child if he is upset (obviously, if he quiets or falls asleep during this time, stay the hell out of the room). When you enter, try not to turn on lights. If lighting is necessary, use a very dim or baby-sleep-friendly bulb that will not inspire wakefulness. Light inhibits specific sleep-promoting pathways in the brain that will be discussed at length later. For now, just try to keep things dark. Additionally, try not to use food to console your child either as you do not want to establish this time as a feeding time. Food is a great way to entrain the circadian rhythm. The last thing we want to do is to "teach" your child's brain to expect food at the precise time you are trying to get him to sleep. Once your child settles (not once your child falls asleep), replace him back in his crib/bed and try again. Don't forget to reset your timer. Again, it's perfectly okay to pop in on older kids and offer words of reassurance.

Settle in. You may be doing this for a while. I cannot impress upon you how important it is to expect to be busy for the next few hours (days? weeks?). Maybe instead of sitting down to figure out some complicated *Good Will Hunting* math equation, you put on an episode of *Real Housewives*. Who cares if the episode gets interrupted? Interrupting the melodrama might actually feel like a good thing.

In my experience, this is where the whole process fails. A parent has been with their child all day and wants—nay deserves—a break. As they allow themselves to look forward to this period of respite, the anticipation of the quiet, relaxed evening sets the stage for the crushing disappointment of how the night is really going to go. Do not let yourself go there. That time of quiet will come, but that time is not right now.

As days pass, start gradually extending the period of time you stay outside his room. Even adding an additional thirty seconds is meaningful.

This process goes on as long as it takes. Usually at the one-hour mark, many parents will say "Screw this," bring the baby into bed with them, and then the following morning write a nasty review of the parenting book on Amazon saying, "This book doesn't work." This process is not easy, especially if you need to work the next day!

As the night mercifully comes to an end and you reach your child's wake time, SLEEP IS OVER. This can be an incredibly hard thing to enforce if you have not gotten sleep during the night. This is where you might need to employ the help of others temporarily. It is essential that if your child did not sleep well during the night, he not be allowed to sleep during the day outside his scheduled naps, and those naps need to be established and stuck to as well. Remember your schedule? It is easy to allow your child to sleep beyond the time of his nap termination, especially if you are using the time to catch up on your own sleep or trying to get other things done.

As time passes, your child will begin to understand that you are always nearby, and sleep will come in larger and larger blocks.

Limit-Setting Disorder

The aforementioned is all well and good for a child who has not acquired the necessary skills for removing himself from his bed (or crib!). They can scream, protest, and moan, but they are at least locked into one location and unable to enter your bedroom and spread their wakeful terrorism. What about an ambulatory sleep disaster?

When a child achieves the ability to move around prior to gaining the gift of reason, we've got trouble. My oldest son began walking very early. We were made aware of this itinerant problem one night while my wife and I were enjoying some quiet time and heard a loud thump originating in his bedroom. Subsequent investigation revealed that our one-year-old had climbed out of his crib and was freely roaming around his room.

To paint a more complete picture, what we now had was a child capable enough to escape from his bed but without even the most rudimentary communication skills with which to convey to him that his newfound ability was really cramping Mommy and Daddy's idyllic existence.

That night, we repeatedly placed him back into his crib, only to find that the speed with which he was able to climb out of his crib was increasing. It did not take long to figure out that we were basically training him to torture us. After much thought we decided to make his crib into a "fun tent." We found a lightweight knitted blanket and draped it across the top of the crib like a roof, tying it securely at each corner. Eventually he found he could escape this arrangement as well. By this time, my wife had purchased an interesting tentlike structure online that one could construct on top of the crib. I think the intention of the product was to keep pets out, not kids in. It worked really well for a while, and he seemed genuinely excited to unzip the flap and climb in (we had given in at this point and allowed him to literally scale his crib to enter at night). He honestly had the look of a first-time home buyer.

"Nighty-night!"

Zip.

The tent era lasted several weeks before he began to wiggle his finger into the small hole behind the zipper and work the flap open from the inside. We heard the thump. We made plans to buy a bed.

I'm not going to lie to you, reader. This time period is hard. I'm not sure why parents get so competitive about how early their kids walk. At that point in my life, I did not want my kid to start walking until the few days leading up to preschool. Early walking without rational thought, reason, and clear communication is nightmarish. Kids getting out of bed . . . kids roaming around your home . . . kids waking you up . . . it is all rotten. If you are a single parent and shouldering this responsibility yourself, bless you!

So, how do we get a child to stay in his room and go to bed? This intervention speaks to the heart of *limit-setting disorder.* When children are young, we have complete control of when they are put in their crib, and until they become ambulatory, they are powerless to go anywhere. As children mature and the crib gives way to the bed, behaviors can begin to appear that shave off important sleep time. One more bedtime story. One more potty attempt. One more sweep of the closet and area under the bed for scary things like clowns, monsters, or monster clowns. These behaviors, coupled with parental inability and or frank unwillingness to replace the bars of the crib with new deterrents is limit-setting disorder.*

Kids can become masters of bedtime stalling. It is important to deal with this firmly and appropriately to keep it from getting out of hand and limiting time in bed. The stalling not only reduces time for sleep, but it often creates a stressful transition from wake time to sleep time as the night ends with irritation and frustration on the part of the parent, which works against a peaceful bedtime.

To deal with children who test the boundaries of your patience at night, always be thinking about the schedule you have created. Is the bedtime appropriate or too early? For some children, their behaviors stem from being asked to go to bed a bit earlier than they are ready. Keep this in mind as you adjust your schedule over time.

Prior to bed, stick to an evening routine that has a lot of "mile markers" leading up to bedtime. In other words, after dinner, make sure they know that it is warm bath, then stories, then bedtime at the designated time. After bath, remind them that it is stories, then bedtime. These reminders will keep your child from being "surprised by bedtime." Even for older children and teens (and adults for that matter), ritual leading up to bed is a positive.

And speaking of positive, make your child's bed and bedroom (or sleeping space if they share a room) fun. Remember that the American Academy of Pediatrics does not recommend stuffed animals in bed with your little one until she turns one. If your child is of age, consider special toys or stuffed items that are really inviting. Feel free to reserve some of those friends for only the bed. I've seen beds that are fashioned like late-model Corvettes or look like castles. If sheets and pillows or wall decals with all the Marvel superheroes make your child's bed more fun and you are able, buy them!

---

* To be clear, while this is generally the domain of the two- to three-year-old, "One more video game" or "Five more minutes on FaceTime with my girlfriend" can be seen in a much older population.

Dealing Effectively with Stalling and Awakenings

Once they are in bed, let your child know that while it is okay to get out of bed, it is not okay to leave the bedroom unless there is something really wrong (fire, intruder, locust swarm, etc.).

When your child does come out of his bedroom or awakens you at night, it is important for you to keep your cool.* Now is the time to keep stress low. Exhibiting a facade that says *Your behavior does not bother me* is important, because kids are opportunistic creatures, and they will exploit your weaknesses. Project an image that you are totally unfazed . . . even bored by the whole affair.† Another tactic is to be honest with your child and tell her that waking you up makes you feel "grumpy" or that waking up Mommy makes you sad or "hurts my feelings." It is important that the child know that the act is hurtful to you. One of my favorite questions to ask kids in my clinic is "Why do you wake up Mommy at night and make her tired? Do you think she can make you fall asleep?" The looks and responses to this are priceless. I have suggested to some parents that when they are awakened by their kids at night, they make a show of pretending to be upset or sad, and it is often highly effective. Kids do not seem to mind if their behaviors make you *mad or angry*, but they often have a much stronger aversion to making you *sad*.

In keeping with the low-stress environment, a low interest-level environment is helpful as well. As kids come out needing a fresh cup of water, let them find you doing mind-numbingly mundane tasks. Underneath your child's behaviors is likely a worry that they are missing out on fun stuff at night. When they come out of the room and see the TV off and you "just watching the ceiling fan," it will help diminish their FOMO.‡ If

---

* No abberant response to their behaviors!

† It is like when the movie hostage says, "Whatever they are paying you, I'll double it," and the villain looks completely unfazed by the offer to double his investment. That's the character you are portraying tonight.

‡ For added punch, turn the ceiling fan off when you pretend to watch it.

you need to be with your child, be boring as hell. Interact minimally. Make sure most toys are hidden, and keep a box of "night toys" handy. What are night toys, you ask? Night toys are a sad collection of any toys your kids have broken, outgrown, or have become otherwise disinterested in.

If your child is a little older and particularly stubborn, institute "night adventures." What's a night adventure? When your child comes into your room at 3:00 a.m. try this dialogue:

Huh? What time is it? It is three o'clock in the morning. . . . Are you okay? Oh, you are. What do you want? You just woke up and decided to come into my bedroom and wake me up too? Okay. Well since you're here, I need some help with something. Are you interested? Great. Tonight, I need to go downstairs and help all the lost daddy longlegs get out of the corners in the garage and back home to their families outside. I'm so glad I have someone to do it with. Mommy is asleep, so she doesn't get to come. Let's go! This will be fun.

The reason why I chose this night adventure is because this particular child of mine was not crazy about spiders. He was even less crazy about them when I handed him a headlamp because "we didn't want to wake the spiders up suddenly." Choose the activity carefully. It should not be fun or exciting, but it should not be traumatizing either.* You are just looking for something a bit less inviting than simply staying in bed.

So here we are . . . my son and I heading into the garage, brush and small dustpan in hand with headlamps glowing red on our heads. The headlamps served two purposes. One, it just made the night adventure feel that much more adventure-y. More important, I did not want to unnecessarily expose him to bright light, which would negatively affect his sleep drive. Amid sleepy protests, we managed to brush a few spiders onto dustpans and free them outside. Again, it is important to make the

---

* If I had to choose one for me personally, it would be analyzing paint swatches for the guest bathroom. Feel free to use that one if appropriate to your situation.

entire process relatively neutral (not negative though), but not necessarily fun. Let them know how pleased you are that they are with you. Nowhere in the conversation should it be talked about how they need to stay in their bed.

When the adventure draws to an end, bring the kid back upstairs, tuck him in, and remind him that all he needs to do to have another wonderful night adventure is to simply come into your bedroom when he awakens and wake you up. It is just that easy. My son and I only went on one spider-oriented night adventure. Hopefully yours will too. If this does not work for your child, other activities to consider might be cleaning toilets, recycling sorting, or extra math practice.

The Importance of the Awakening

One way or another, the night plays out and the designated wake time arrives. This wake time represents an important shift from sleep to wakefulness, and your brain pays a lot of attention to this event as many things are happening in a relatively brief window of time:

1. The eyes go from being in the dark to ideally being in light.

2. The body goes from a cool bedroom environment to warm.

3. The body goes from being motionless, at times paralyzed, to being in motion.

4. The individual goes from being solitary to being socially interactive.

5. The gut goes from being in a fasted state to being fed.

These state changes represent dramatic shifts for our nervous system and form the core components of what your child's brain uses to set its sleep/wake cycle and circadian rhythm. These cues are sometimes referred to as zeitgebers (German for "time giver") and they are very important for your child. While paying attention to these zeitgebers is important for everyone, regardless of age, it is even more important to pay attention to them with your young child, as doing so will potentially set the foundation for a lifetime of good sleep.

Light

Every time your child wakes up, she needs to transition from a very dark environment to a very bright one during that set wake-up time. This is particularly important if you live in a dark or dreary place.* Many parents like to establish a quietly lit room for their kids. Quietly lit is great *prior* to bedtime, but rubbish *after* wake time. Turn on those lights . . . all of them, not just the cute little fairy lights you had mounted all over her room. Better yet, open a window. Raising your kids in Fairbanks, Alaska? No problem—buy a light box and set it at the end of your changing table near baby's head. When sleep time is over, stroll into the nursery all smiles, turn on some lights and the light box, scoop up the baby, freshen up his nether region while that light box makes the room bright, and move on with your day! Have older kids? Don't let them disappear into the dark basement dungeon to play *Minecraft*. Force them to spend time in well-lit environments. With their wake periods full of light, it will make your kids much more responsive to the lack of light before bed, helping them fall asleep more quickly.

Temperature

Manipulating temperature in your child's environment can be remarkably helpful in terms of organizing sleep at any age. The great part about it is that it requires no input or even awareness from your child.† There is often discussion about temperature and sleep, but it is usually limited to bedtime. Yes, having your child sleep in a cool environment (65°F or so) can be very helpful in terms of sleep initiation and quality, but do not

* Go Seahawks! God save the Queen! etc.

† I do think that as a child matures, sharing with her the science of temperature and sleep and the reasons for the cooler temperatures at night and warmer temperatures during the day can be confidence boosting in the sleep department and set the stage for good habits as they get older.

stop the temperature considerations there. You've got twenty-four hours to think about. Temperature manipulations around the clock will be discussed at length in chapter 8. Until then, you might want to pick up one of those programmable thermostats like Google Nest makes and set it up to drop the temperature in your home/kid's room around dinnertime to get him ready for sleep.

Food

Food is an easy one. Starting the day off with food at that consistent wake time is important for establishing a positive sleep routine. As with temperature, think about your child's meals around the clock and work to keep them consistent. Big meals prior to bedtime for any child old enough to gorge themselves is not ideal, as it could interfere with both sleep onset and sleep continuity.

Exercise

Get going in the morning. When your kids are small, plop them into the jog stroller and hit the road. As kids get older, strongly encourage them to begin the day with some form of exercise. It can be brief. A simple treadmill jog or dog walk can do the trick. Want to insulate your children from sleep problems the rest of their lives? Sign them up for morning swim team. Even if they have basketball practice later in the day, the burst of activity (and the body temperature bump that goes along with it) can be extremely impactful to their sleep the upcoming night.

Social Interaction

Remember when we were talking about kids who got up too early or woke up in the night, and I said to be really boring when you interact with them? Here is the reason why. Social interaction is a cue for wakefulness. Do not let your teen skulk out of his room and down to the basement in the morning. Greet him! Force him to sit and have breakfast with you. Better yet, force him to walk the dog with you! Outside light (☐), warmer temperature (☐), activity (☐), and social interaction (☐). There's absolutely no better way to start the day.

One morning, Charlie and his mother are walking the dog on a street in his neighborhood. When I video chatted Mom, she said what a lot of parents say to me. "What you said about Charlie's sleep made sense and gave me hope. I was in such a bad place when I saw you. Even just hearing you say 'Charlie sleeps' empowered me. My husband and I totally changed our attitudes and language about Charlie and his sleep, and I was shocked by how quickly things changed."

While her words were positive, the two weeks it took to get to this place were not a walk in the park. Charlie did not give up the ship easily, but eventually he did. They all do.

When Charlie came back for a follow-up visit, it was abundantly clear that he was proud of himself and his sleep. It was also apparent that there was a new sheriff in town when Charlie reached into his mother's purse for the phone and she merely looked at him sternly and he put it back.

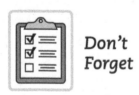 Don't
Forget

1. A huge determinant of your child's sleep quality is his schedule. Keep in mind, the sleep need of kids is changing constantly, so the schedule will need to be updated accordingly.

2. Understand the proper definition of a bedtime, and that wake times don't vary.

3. Be patient and set the proper tone when kids test bedtime boundaries.

4. Have a plan for handling unwanted awakenings and children who invite themselves into your bedroom at night.

5

Insufficient-Sleep Disorders
and School Start Times

How to Find a School Bus in the Dark

 Zoe is a thirteen-year-old girl with purple hair that makes Ziggy Stardust's red mullet look bland and colorless. She seems genuinely thrilled to be in my office and is one of those kids who can do the whole visit herself. All she needs is a ride. She has come to the clinic with her mother, who is concerned about Zoe's sleepiness.

Zoe's mother (Angel) gave birth to Zoe when she was in a committed relationship with another woman. As such, Zoe lives with Angel, but does spend some amount of visitation time with her other mother. During the time Zoe is with Angel, there are many moving parts to the schedule, mostly related to Angel's work and which adult is taking care of Zoe. Currently, the responsibility for Zoe's care falls to one of the following:

- Angel
- Angel's current committed partner

- Zoe's other mother

- Zoe's grandmother

- Zoe's school

The coordination of these five entities is no simple task and often requires Zoe to awaken early on a school day to be dropped off at her grandmother's home so that Angel can get to her job on days she has to be there early. Because of the proximity of Angel's home to her mother's and to her job, Zoe is forced to get up very early on these days . . . two or three times per week.

Unfortunately, Zoe's sleep gets squeezed from the other end as well, as Angel is quite the roller derby queen, and Zoe goes along with Angel to practice. Zoe, an amateur photographer, proudly shows me some outstanding action shots of twenty- to fiftysomething-year-old women bashing each other in a local convention center turned roller derby rink. The practices typically run on the later side to accommodate the work schedules of those involved.

"What happens on days that you are at the derby practice at night and have to go to your grandmother's house the next morning?"

Zoe looks to her mother as a defendant might look to her attorney before answering a difficult question.

"Those mornings are hard. Zoe has an 'early bird' jazz band class that starts at seven forty-five, but she does okay. Fortunately, Zoe is good at making up the sleep on the weekends."

~ ~ ~

As a child grows up, she will face a constant barrage of obstacles working to prevent her from achieving adequate sleep. Permissive parents, school schedules, homework policies, extracurricular activities, and laptops or phones in the bedroom at night all represent extrinsic threats to children and teenagers getting the sleep they need. While the majority of this book looks inward at the conditions that affect children's sleep, this chapter explores the external obstacles to healthy sleep.

Zoe is not alone. The numbers are epidemic-level and shocking. A recent abstract presented at the 2019 American Academy of Pediatrics national conference calculated that 52 percent of children in the six-to-seventeen age group are getting eight hours of sleep or fewer. Lead author Hoi See Tsao, MD, a pediatrician in Boston, analyzed survey data from 49,050 subjects prior to concluding that this insufficient amount of sleep was preventing these children from flourishing both in and out of school. Moving up to high school students, the numbers are truly staggering. In 2018, the Centers for Disease Control and Prevention (CDC) issued a report estimating that two out of every three high school adolescents are not getting eight hours of sleep or more on school nights, the number they deemed to be sufficient.

I placed this chapter after the insomnia chapter for a reason, and it is an important one. I want to illustrate and contrast the differences between insomnia and sleep deprivation, because in the minds of many, they are synonymous. They are not. If the previous chapter about insomnia was about kids who feel they "can't sleep," think of the kids in this chapter as the ones who "won't sleep," or in many cases are not given adequate opportunity to do so.

 Historically, not allowing or facilitating adequate sleep in children was not looked upon favorably. Anna Steese Richardson had some strong words for parents like Angel who allowed their kids to stay up too late.

Nature cries out for sleep. Parents interfere with nature by starting the baby off wrong and teaching it not to want sleep. The best argument is that the baby who is kept up to romp with Papa in the evening at age two, three, or four years, is a late sleeper in the morning, irritable, and heavy.

Papa just got burned. Back in the day, it was the mother's absolute responsibility to ensure that her children had ample, consistent, and uninterrupted time for sleep, and that if the milkman needed to make a delivery, he'd better be damn quiet about the whole affair, lest an "irritable" mother take a broom handle to his "heavy" backsides.

What Is Inadequate Sleep in Children?

More than one hundred years later, we still have not stopped talking about sleep need and the importance of getting adequate rest. One of the awesome things about sleep science is that it is in the media at a near constant level.

Just look through the magazines in the checkout aisles the next time you're at the grocery store; there will always be a cover mention about sleep. In truth, I love the idea that the public has an interest and enthusiasm for sleeping better. Suddenly the population has stopped viewing sleep as a fixed trait and now sees sleep as a modifiable variable in their lives. That's wonderful!

Despite being a positive, the fact that sleep science is constantly in the media can also be a big negative. With such a heavy output of sleep headlines across all media, messages and information can get a bit twisted, and in particular the messages about "insomnia" and the messages about inadequate sleep or "sleep deprivation."

We have already extensively explored the ideas of insomnia in the previous chapter, and in particular the problems with sleep efficiency, sleep predictability, and sleep perception. It is worth noting that at no point in that chapter did we talk about: (1) sleep deprivation, or (2) any tragic health consequences that go along with insomnia. This relates to a sleep mentor's comment to me when I was early in my training—"Insomnia is the worst condition in the world that has virtually no medical consequence."

Contrast insomnia with sleep deprivation. Imagine your daughter in the throes of midterms her junior year of high school. Studying, cramming, working into the night to try to complete difficult essays and prepare herself for tough exams. What happens when she finally finishes her final test and turns in that last paper? She comes home and crashes for fourteen hours straight. This is what sleep deprivation looks like.

And sleep deprivation is harmful. Very harmful. Intentionally depriving oneself of sleep is a hazardous activity for all kinds of reasons. It can affect memory, mood, immune system functioning, normal growth and maturation, heart health, academic and athletic performance, attention, and even tendencies for certain cancers. In other words, sleep deprivation is slowly shortening your life (weight gain, high blood pressure) while simultaneously trying to end it quickly (car accident, stroke).

And herein lies the problem with the media's portrayal of sleep and how it shapes our public's (and children's, and medical community's) understanding of sleep. Basically, there are two main headlines we are exposed to regarding sleep:

1. Tips and strategies for people (adults and kids alike) who "can't sleep."

2. The health and performance consequences of not sleeping (scary!).

Now consider those two main headlines. Do you see the natural connection that most people make?

If my child cannot sleep (#1) . . . bad things will happen (#2).

Knowing everything you know about sleep at this point, you can probably see what's wrong with this statement. It is the word "cannot." If there is one thing you should take away from this book, it is that sleep is inevitable. The media does not do a good job of making it clear that the articles about kids not sleeping (sleep deprivation) are aimed at a totally different audience than the articles aimed at the parents whose kids have trouble falling asleep (insomnia). To make this a true statement, the relationship should read:

If a child chooses not to acquire adequate sleep, or is not given adequate time to sleep, bad things will happen.

But because this isn't made clear to parents, this leads to bad conclusions and often unhelpful or even harmful actions taken to fix the problem. Here is one common path a parent goes down:

"My child, like all kids, needs sleep to be healthy."
I totally agree!
"I've read a lot about how a child who gets an inadequate amount
    of sleep is at increased risk for health and performance problems
    and other serious consequences. Yikes."

Yes! I know. Sleep is supremely important.

"My son really struggles to fall asleep. Sometimes it takes him
  hours."

I'm sorry to hear that, maybe he should . . .

"I warn him every night that if he doesn't fall asleep faster and get
  more sleep, he's going to get Alzheimer's disease and not get
  into a good college."

Whoa, back up there a bit, I'm not sure . . .

"No, it is true. That TV doctor said so. He also mentioned some
  homeopathic vitamins supplements I can buy that . . ."

And if you've been paying attention, you can see where that parent
went wrong. I want you to move into this chapter with a clear vision of
your child. Keep in mind that children can experience the symptoms of
both insomnia and sleep deprivation simultaneously. *They are by no means
mutually exclusive.*

Symptoms of Sleep Deprivation

For most children, the most consistent sign of sleep deprivation is excessive daytime sleepiness (EDS). Excessive daytime sleepiness is exactly as
it sounds—a child who is exhibiting a strong drive to sleep during the
day, or time in which he should be awake. Think of it as a brain seeking
sleep because the amount it received at night was not enough to satisfy
its need.

Generally, EDS is easy to spot. Think of a mother falling asleep during
her kid's school production of *West Side Story.** While Mom's sleepiness
is obvious, spotting inadequate sleep in kids is not always so easy. Young
kids often do not manifest excessive daytime sleepiness in the same way
adults do. We often say that children seem to "spiral up" when they are
sleepy. Instead of the classic sleepy guy in a long college lecture, eyes
heavy, head bobbing, sometimes quite dramatically, kids can seem hyper
and overexcited. Perhaps they run naked through the house with their

---

* In Mom's defense on that one, her kid was Jet #3, and as such did not have the most
wake-promoting part, although he really did his best in "Jet Song."

underwear on their heads like hats, laughing hysterically. Hardly the grandpa-sleeping-in-the-La-Z-Boy look. For children, sleepiness is often an uncomfortable feeling they want to fight. Their sleepiness can often make them moody, irrational, and inattentive with significant deficits in emotional regulation. This is why symptoms of extreme sleepiness are often overlooked. The last word some parents would use to describe these kids would be "sleepy."

Diagnosing Inadequate Sleep in Children

So how does one go about evaluating their child for inadequate sleep and the often-occurring excessive daytime sleepiness? For infants and very young children, it can be hard. Babies sleep a lot. A sleeping baby is not typically something that many people will question too aggressively.

As children mature and there is a natural reduction in sleep need, inadequate sleep may be easier to spot. Comparisons with other children or conversations with other parents or teachers may suggest that your child is sleeping too much outside the designated sleep window. Is your child seeking sleep either intentionally or inadvertently during normal waking hours? Is she falling asleep in unusual places (in the shopping cart while you're buying groceries, on the bench during a baseball game)? If there are concerns, there are some validated assessments to help you determine the degree of your child's sleepiness.

One assessment commonly used to evaluate sleepiness is the Epworth Sleepiness Scale for Children and Adolescents (ESS-CHAD). While it has been validated only for kids twelve to eighteen, even in ages outside that range, it can still serve as a useful tool to get the ball rolling!

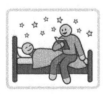 Here is how it works. If you think your child is capable of answering some simple questions, give them the following scenarios. Ask them to imagine themselves in these eight situations, and determine how likely it would be for them to fall asleep.

EPWORTH SLEEPINESS SCALE—CHAD

Situation	Would never fall asleep	Slight chance of falling asleep	Moderate chance of falling asleep	High chance of falling asleep
Sitting and reading	0	1	2	3
Watching TV or a video	0	1	2	3
Sitting in a classroom at school during the morning	0	1	2	3
Sitting and riding in a car or bus for about half an hour	0	1	2	3
Lying down to rest or nap in the afternoon	0	1	2	3
Sitting and talking to someone	0	1	2	3
Sitting quietly by yourself after lunch	0	1	2	3
Sitting and eating a meal	0	1	2	3

Once you have answered the questions, simply tabulate the numerical sum of the answers, and you now have your kid's ESS-CHAD score. How did she do? Interpreting the results is easy: scores ten and above indicate excessive daytime sleepiness.

The ESS-CHAD is a powerful tool. While I'm introducing it in this chapter, it can be useful throughout this book (and in the assessment of your children) to screen for an artificially high drive to sleep. It does not differentiate between intrinsic and extrinsic causes . . . only whether sleepiness exists. The nice thing about the scale is that it is completely objective. As an example, a parent who is a sound sleeper may be totally in the dark about his child staying up too late. This study does not rely on the detection of the behavior (or disorder) . . . just its consequence.

There are lots of potential causes of excessive sleepiness in a child. I like to divide them into intrinsic and extrinsic causes.

Intrinsic (poor quality)	Extrinsic (poor quantity)
Sleep apnea	Stalling prior to bed (limit-setting)
Acid reflux	Early school start times
Restless legs	Heavy workload and/or extracurricular schedule
Nocturnal seizures	Noisy bedroom / electronics / poor sleep hygiene

Much of this book is devoted to the specific intrinsic causes of excessive sleepiness. Often, the diagnoses are found and treated only because a parent observed excessive sleepiness in their child, despite adequate sleep, and started asking questions! Each of these causes will be dealt with specifically in their own chapter. This chapter focuses mainly on the extrinsic or environmental causes of inadequate sleep.

Let's start with the basics. The first question to ask when a child is displaying signs of excessive daytime sleepiness is simple. Is your child getting enough rest? A basic lack of sleep quantity will almost universally lead your child to display signs of excessive daytime sleepiness. Does your child stay up too late reading or watching television? Children of divided families are particularly at risk of staying up too late, as shown by University of Pennsylvania researcher Brittany Rudd's 2019 investigation of divided families and the impact on sleep. A child may be going to bed on time in one home, but permitted to remain awake in the partner's residence. This permissive behavior is a way parents attempt to gain favor with children. In fact, studies show that television and portable electronics are the number one factor in children getting inadequate sleep. I am doubtful that this is particularly earth-shattering news. If you feel like your daughter's incessant need to read ahead in her statistics class is the main issue, you might be an outlier here.

I do not think it is necessary to beat this topic to death. Is your child showing signs of excessive sleepiness? Is your child spending too little time in bed? I think you know what the intervention is . . . an earlier bedtime and more sleep. If you can make this happen easily, great. Do it and skip to the end of this chapter.

But telling a parent they just need to get their kids to sleep more is a bit like telling someone that the solution to their obesity is simple—just lose weight. Perfectly easy to say and almost impossible at times to achieve.

To me, the obstacles preventing your child from getting adequate sleep are like the levels of a video game. Level one is simply trying to get your new baby on some kind of schedule that makes sense. It is the first level of *Donkey Kong*. A little tough initially, but once you figure out how the barrels roll, it is pretty easy to master.

Subsequent levels are not as easy. As your child begins to mature, stalling before bed and fighting sleep are common. The limit-setting strategies we covered in the previous chapter are essential for helping to mold sleepers who seek adequate time in bed. Again, these issues are pretty self-limited if parents can maintain some kind of schedule regularity.

The next level(s) relate(s) to school, and suddenly much of the control over your child's schedule is taken out of your hands. In my opinion, school is the clearest and most present threat to your child getting a healthy amount of sleep. If the COVID crisis has taught us anything, it is the fact that the removal of a rigid, in-person school schedule has resulted in a dramatic increase in sleep time for many children.* Dr. Bobbi Hopkins, pediatric neurologist and medical director of the Johns Hopkins All Children's Sleep Clinic recently said, "These kids are sleeping longer; closer to the recommended amount of sleep because they have time to do so."

---

* For my kids, the increase has been profound. The delay of school start times and the removal of early-morning swimming and rowing practice has made the change even more remarkable. While it is only the results of two kids, both of my boys (ages fifteen and eighteen) began growing more rapidly during this time. While access to a refrigerator all day long could be the explanation, I choose to believe that the enhanced growth hormone secretion accompanying the increase in deep sleep acquisition is the cause.

Schools and Sleep

Within the topic of school, there are many subjects I want to tackle: school start times, how schools tend to favor children who deal better with sleep deprivation than others, and weekday versus weekend schedules.

School Start Times

School start times are a current and ongoing topic of great debate. You may be aware of (or participating in) the debate where your child or children go to school. The debate hypothesis is simple:

Schools start too early and are negatively impacting the amount of sleep our children are able to get during the school year. This sleep deprivation is adversely impacting their health and school performance.

That sounds simple and logical enough. The counterargument goes something like this:

If schools start later, kids will simply stay up later, negating the effects of the delayed start time. Furthermore, the disruption to parent work schedules, the busing of kids, and after-school activities like sports make the changes difficult if not impossible to implement.

This debate is not new. It's been a topic slowly gaining momentum and data for several years. If you simply look at school start times, the data is clear:

- Kids sleep more when school start times are delayed. They do not simply use the time to stay up later. I suspect there will be many studies that come out of the COVID-19 pandemic further amplifying this principle.

- School performance and health measures improve with later school start times. Studies have shown improvements in academic performance across the entire school day, less absenteeism, and even less drug use in children who start the day later.

- The Hamilton Project (an economic policy initiative within the Brookings Institute) estimated in 2011 that middle school students would earn $17,500 more over their lifetime if school start times were delayed one hour. Even outcomes like car crashes have been shown to happen more frequently in early-morning driving in kids. The Hamilton Project concluded that economically, the reasons for delaying start times outnumbered the reasons for keeping things as is, nine to one.

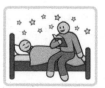 School and Sleep Deprivation
In a bubble, the choice for starting schools later would be simple. The problem is the logistics. Altering school start times is difficult, highly political, and predicated on far more criteria than simply student health and performance. Let's forget that, and focus on your child by reviewing some simple statements related to school start times:

SCHOOL START TIME CHECKLIST

❐ My child seems to show signs of excessive daytime sleepiness.

❐ My child is consistently getting an inadequate amount of sleep.

❐ My child's school begins at 8:30 a.m. or earlier.

❐ My child has a bus ride that exceeds thirty minutes one way.

❐ My child sleeps an additional two hours more on the weekends.

❐ My child struggles with issues of mood and behavior.

If you checked off two or more of these statements, I think it is reasonable to consider your child's school as a potential problem when it comes to adequate sleep. Asking these difficult questions matters, as studies have shown that not only can early school start times impact a child's academic performance in their early-morning classes, but they can also negatively impact performance for their entire school day.

From the first day your son rides away on the bus for kindergarten all the way to college, parents must be vigilant in monitoring their child's sleep needs.* As your child matures, school becomes much more labor intensive, and at the same time, the stakes become higher. Color outside the lines as a first grader . . . that can probably be explained away during a job interview later. Botch an AP calculus class as a high school senior . . . not so easy to sweep under the rug. As kids grow up, it becomes just as important to evaluate the school and schedule itself as it does how your child navigates it.

Recognizing sleepiness is difficult. We've established that in a young kid, but what about older students? A high schooler can get home from a swim meet, bang out a final draft of an English essay, and start studying for a government exam at midnight and may not look particularly hampered by fatigue. "As long as I get my four hours, I'm good to go" is the familiar battle cry. And sure enough, they snag two personal records at the swim meet, solid A- on the essay, and while the results of the government exam are not back yet, the feeling is that it went really well.

The ability of a child to stay up late and succeed in school is often looked upon as a positive rather than a negative, and this does not end with high school. In residency, we called it horsepower. Who cares how smart a neurology resident is when they are too tired to pull their weight during all-night hospital call? And like so many other things we have talked about in this book, horsepower is genetic.

To understand horsepower, sleep need, and functional levels, consider these three high school students who are only getting an average of 4.5 hours of sleep/night:

* It really doesn't stop then, but your level of involvement/power will most likely be diminished significantly!

	Average Sleep (hours)	Biological Sleep Need (hours)	Horsepower Gene	Short Sleeper Gene	Functional Level
Kourtney	4.5	7	no	no	poor
Kim	4.5	7	yes	no	excellent
Khloé	4.5	4.5	no	yes	excellent

If we consider Kourtney, we see that while she needs seven hours of sleep, she is only getting an average of 4.5 hours every night. She does not have the gene allowing for high function despite inadequate sleep (horsepower), so she functions poorly and struggles to stay awake in school.

Kim too is only sleeping 4.5 hours per night despite needing seven, but she was given the gift of the horsepower gene, and despite inadequate rest, she functions at a high level. The horsepower gene may be a genetic variant of HLA DQB1*0602, the gene related to narcolepsy. Individuals with this gene variant may find less sleepiness as a consequence of sleep deprivation. While this state of sleep deprivation is still an unhealthy situation for Kim, she does not display significant sleepiness. In other words, it's totally unhealthy, but Kim can handle it!

Last, in this example we see Khloé too is only getting 4.5 hours of sleep every night, but this is in line with her natural biological need, which seems on the surface to be unusually low. She functions well despite a lower than average amount of sleep because this is what she requires . . . no need for the horsepower gene to help her perform well if her perceived deficit is not really a deficit.

You may remember a name for people like Khloé. We call them *short sleepers*. They are those individuals who need less than normal amounts of sleep to function at their best. Once again, let's look back at the NSF graph for sleep need (page 13). Notice how there are no age categories that show 4.5 hours within the range of normal.* Despite this, Khloé is doing well because she genetically needs less sleep.

The genetic basis for these rare, rule-defying individuals was only re-

---

* This is true for older age groups as well. The oldest age group of older adult (sixty-five years and older) lists five to six hours as the lowest range of normal.

cently discovered when specific gene mutations regulating sleep need were identified.

The point of explaining all this to you is that your child is a totally unique individual with a specific array of genes that this world has never and will never see again. It is important to constantly be evaluating their sleep time and functional level. If they are getting the requisite amount of sleep and functioning well, there is little that needs to be done outside of ongoing monitoring. If your child is not getting the proper amount and is not functioning well, he may need more. As we see with Khloé, Kim, and Kourtney, for the child functioning well getting what appears to be a small amount of sleep, it may be necessary to insist upon more sleep and see if your child utilizes the sleep time (a Kim, so to speak) or seems incapable of getting this new higher amount (the rare Khloé).

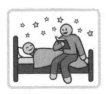

Treating Inadequate Sleep in Children

Your child is not getting enough sleep. Given that this is a very heterogenous topic, the way the problem is addressed can take many forms. Hopefully at this point, your child has a schedule that is fairly firm and has established sleep habits.

We've already discussed how school is the most likely cause of inadequate sleep, and it's not a problem that can be solved with a sticker chart. To adequately address school, multiple layers of the situation need to be evaluated.

First, is the school's schedule (including busing, if appropriate) conducive to an optimal resting situation? To determine this, examine what time your child must be awake to get on the school bus to go to school and when school begins. The American Academy of Pediatrics says schools should begin at 8:30 a.m. or later, and commonly thirty minutes or less is cited as an appropriate one-way bus ride. If your child's school start time is earlier than 8:30 a.m., their bus trip is prolonged, or both, contacting the school may be necessary. Find out if your school district has an organized group fighting to improve this issue. If not, visit the National Sleep Foundation or Start School Later (www.startschoollater .net) for ways to effect change in your school district.

Start times are really just the beginning of the fight. What's the use of a healthy start time if students are so burdened by work they can't make use of the time to sleep? To me, this is where school issues begin to get very difficult. My oldest daughter (big horsepower) often argues that, with college and graduate school on the horizon, kids need to learn how to deal with sleep deprivation. At the risk of this exploding into a great philosophical debate about the heartiness of our culture and its value on sleep, I agree that she probably has a point. That said, I personally believe that many young children are being forced to sacrifice sleep in order to excel academically or athletically.

And so, looking beyond school, it is time to evaluate your student and what she can do to improve the situation.

Question #1: Is your child overscheduled? Fair warning. Once again, we are moving a bit away from Dr. Winter, sleep expert, and more toward Chris Winter, random vocal parent of some kids at a school. Have you ever gone to a restaurant and ordered an entrée and then been caught off guard by the waiter when he says that you get two sides with your order? Then you look down at the bottom of the menu and there's all kinds of items like fries, steamed vegetables, or jalapeño creamed corn with bacon. It is my personal opinion that *every* child should be able to attend school (the entrée) and still be able to choose two of the following "sides":

play a sport
play a musical instrument
participate in a hobby or club like painting, Scouts, robotics team
volunteer
be active in a religious youth group (Young Life, B'nai B'rith, etc.)
dance
sing

I can't quite bring myself to put "play video games" on here, but . . .

It frustrates me when I feel like "school" does not allow for the development of the whole child, because said child is getting slammed with homework and other school responsibilities. Therefore, I think every child has a right to participate in at least two extracurricular activities. Can your child do three or four? Sure, but I think those become privileges, not rights. In other words, if your child can handle it, do well in school, and get her requisite sleep, go for it. If your child cannot, all I'm saying is I cannot defend the decision you are making; I'm going to recommend that one or two of the activities need to go.

Your child is playing baseball and is very active in Scouts, which is great. What on earth is standing in her way from having it all? Most likely homework. This was a frequent conversation in my home as our kids grew up.

Monday

"Got a lot of homework, son?"

"Nope . . . no homework or tests."

Tuesday

"Got a lot of homework, son?"

"Nope . . . no homework or tests."

Wednesday

"Got a lot of homework, son?"

"Nope . . . no homework or tests."

Thursday

"Ahhhhhh! I've got three tests tomorrow and a ton of home-work!"

"Well, you should have been studying and keeping up."

"I am, but we just got this assignment today, and nobody knew about the tests."

I know what you are thinking. "Chris, your kids are procrastinating and need to step it up in the work-anticipation category." Believe me, I thought so too. Lots of *How does everyone else know about . . . ?* arguments were had in this house. Over time, and with subsequent children saying the same things, it became clear they were telling the truth. Looking at texts and emails between the students . . . many of them exceptionally bright kids, showed that everyone was in the dark about testing schedules and sudden surges of homework.

Back in my day, this was not a thing. If Ms. Ankrom was giving a calculus exam, Mr. Johnston knew about it and might delay his US History exam a day or two. Likewise, Mrs. Hartenstein would give us an extra day on our *American Tragedy* essay. Teachers were cool back then.

What this means is that you have got to run interference for your kids. While I'm not advocating an adversarial relationship with your kids' school, I'm also not advocating that you just allow your kid to "take it" either. Most schools will tell you, to your face, something like, "If you feel like your child has put the requisite effort and time into homework, you can tell them to go to bed and just send us a note and they will be excused." I'm not sure what the technical word would be for this situation, but in my experience, that is total bullshit. It is like the *I Love Lucy* episode where Lucy and Ethel are working at the chocolate factory. Imagine her boss saying, "Take a break whenever you want, just make sure the chocolates get packaged properly." This plan does not work if the conveyor belt with the chocolate never stops or even slows down. And therein lies the problem. What the principal says has no relation to the conveyor belt the teachers control.*

So unfortunately, this forces many families (ours included) to create "sick days" so our kids can catch up on work missed from a swim meet or dance recital. Not everyone has this luxury, so I'm sure many kids pay a heavy academic price. I often think about this as kids graduate from high school: how many children wearing the rope or stole indicating academic exceptionalism are truly so, and how many just had parents

---

* To be clear, I love teachers. Both my parents were high school teachers. I married a teacher too. I'm not blaming teachers. This is often a systemic problem that upsets and frustrates teachers as much as it does students and parents.

with the means who were able to work behind the scenes to help make that so?

What can be done if your child is organized and disciplined about their studies and activities but still does not always have adequate time for sleep? What if your mother has to drop her daughter off very early during the week in order for everyone to be on time? We have already focused a lot on establishing a consistent sleep schedule for your children, a process that probably started the day they were born. Now, I'm about to suggest something that might feel at odds with this idea.

Sleep Debt

Within the field of sleep medicine is a concept of *sleep debt*. Think of sleep debt as an ongoing tab or credit card related to sleep need. Ideally a child wakes up, accumulates a daily sleep debt or tab, and pays it in full at the end of the day, starting with a clean slate in the morning. And so, the right thing to do with sleep and the right thing to do with a credit card or tab is to pay it in full immediately.*

Sometimes you can't though. The car needs a new transmission and funds are a bit inadequate to cover that expense outright. No problem, that's what the credit card is for. However, a smart consumer is going to make a plan immediately for paying that credit card bill down quickly to avoid unnecessary interest payments and fees. Sometimes a child cannot get their needed sleep because of a soccer game far away that went into overtime and eventually penalty kicks. Sometimes there will be two tests and a paper due on Thursday. What will the plan be under these circumstances?

The answer may be to establish a line of "sleep credit." Recent research has concluded that short-term sleep debts can be paid off with little to no health consequences. It is like those credit deals you get on new appliances. "Buy your new washer and dryer and pay no money down and no interest for the first six months." Boom. Not only can you upgrade to a washing machine that actually cleans clothes and does it quietly, but you

---

* It would be really helpful if along with a child's sleep debt, there was a corresponding "sleep credit rating" that indicated how consistently her sleep debt is being paid.

can spread the expense out over a short period of time with no penalty. Great!

This research says that you can think about sleep in a similar way. If you can't come up with the full amount of sleep necessary, you can pay it back over a short period of time at no cost to your child's health and well-being. The logical follow-up question is, how long? Twenty-four hours? One week? Six months? Longer?

Before I give what I believe the answer to this question is, it's important to note two things: (1) This idea of how long you can go between missed sleep and repaying the sleep debt with interest (e.g., health consequences) is hotly debated among sleep experts, with some saying no debt can be fully repaid, and (2) The evidence is all over the place, so you are getting my take—good or bad. With that disclaimer, in my opinion, I think it is safe to repay a sleep debt within one week. In other words, any sleep loss—borrowed sleep—can be repaid by an individual within a week at no real consequence to their overall health or their chances of leading a long and healthy life. This conclusion is supported by several studies, including a Swedish cohort study evaluating 43,880 subjects.

Stated another way, think of your child's sleep need not as nine hours per night, but rather sixty-three hours per week. Your job is to work with your child to make sure that goal is met, understanding that while consistency is best if at all possible, less consistent sleep will do if necessary.

Now, like any good agreement, there is fine print. This agreement is not a statement that says it is okay for your child to pull consecutive all-nighters and then just sleep all weekend to hit their weekly hour target. There are very real immediate dangers to voluntary sleep deprivation—just think of young drivers. Second, making up the sleep debt sooner rather than later is something most sleep experts would agree is best. Don't wait until the weekend if Monday's difficult night could be made up for by an earlier bedtime on Tuesday. Finally, trying to keep consistency in mind as you make up the sleep is very important. Choosing a slightly earlier bedtime over three nights is much better than a huge four-hour nap on Saturday afternoon that is disruptive to light exposure, meal timing, and exercise on Saturday, and might negatively affect Saturday night's sleep.

While this should never be the basis of an established sleep routine, it can at least be a contingency plan when things go sideways with your child's sleep. Teaching this technique can help to build resiliency and a sense of empowerment when circumstances are outside of their (or your) control.

Armed with a letter from my office, Zoe and her mother were able to reach an agreement with her school that if Zoe was sleepy, she could utilize her study hall and even homeroom period to rest or sleep in the nurse's office. Over the years, I have had many students reach similar agreements with their schools, universities, and even employers. More important, Zoe reached an agreement with her mother that two or three nights per week, bedtime would be moved up thirty minutes to build in an additional hour and a half of sleep into her schedule. After eliminating the phone from the bedroom, Zoe never seemed to have any difficulty falling asleep at that earlier time and reported not only feeling more energetic but also being in a better mood and having better academic performance after the changes. She still takes roller derby pictures.

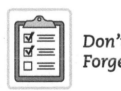

Don't Forget

1. Looking at both the time your child sleeps and resultant behavior, ask yourself the question "Is my child getting enough sleep?"

2. Experiment with adding in extra sleep time at night. Does your child gobble it up, or seem incapable of utilizing it?

3. How are school and extracurricular activities factoring into your child's sleep opportunities? What opportunities exist to shift the balance of sleep time more in your child's favor?

4. In the midst of inescapable sleep conflicts, do you have a plan to repay your child's sleep debt?

Sleep and Disorders of Attention

"Can You Repeat That? I Was Thinking About a Spaceship."

 The setup for most pediatricians' exam rooms is pretty straightforward. Exam table, chairs for parents/spouses/friends/caregivers, a stool or chair with rollers on it for the doctor when she comes in, a sink, some cabinets, a degree or certification on the wall, and some *Highlights* magazines with the Hidden Pictures activity callously circled in pen, ruining it for future readers. It's a relatively basic layout with simple rules for seating. Kid on the table, Mom and/or Dad in the chairs, doctor in the roller seat.

A hint that my patient may have attention deficit hyperactivity disorder (ADHD) often surfaces as soon as I walk into the exam room. Parents are in the chairs with sister on one lap. Brother is in the prone Superman position, belly down on the roller chair, phone in hand, recklessly launching himself across the exam room by pushing off from the walls.* As I walk in, there is no acknowledgment of the chair theft or massive black shoe marks on the walls, but rather a look like, *I deal with this twenty-four hours a day. I think you can handle forty-five minutes.* And I can. And I have Magic Erasers. It is all good.

"Emory, can you give me the phone and stop racing around on the doctor's chair?"

As if that was going to work, but nice show of effort.

For the next hour, a lot of information is communicated in my direction. Emory is ten and has a lot going on both in and out of school. Scholastic struggles, medical conditions, and discipline issues (at some point, there will be a passive-aggressive shot at the other partner about some discipline action or nonaction with the unspoken assumption that I will render a verdict as to which parent is right). The list is long and difficult. These parents are worn out in the deepest, most fundamental sense.

At some point, someone has raised the idea of this child having ADHD and after being around him for only a few minutes (not counting the waiting room), it is not hard to see why. It is a perfectly valid hypothesis.

Fortunately, this child has a pediatrician who is an out-of-the-box thinker and immediately started asking about Emory's sleep. While his sleep seemed disturbed at times, there was no indication from either parent about snoring or any indication of breathing issues. He often got into bed with them, so outside of the annoyance of him "breathing his night breath in our faces," nothing was ever noted to be amiss. Emory did sleep in Pull-Ups until "seven or eight" but was 100 percent dry at night now.

After our evaluation, it boiled down to my personal rule when it comes to kids and ADHD: no child should be diagnosed with ADHD without first having a sleep evaluation. I told them I did not suspect the

---

* Technically, this is actually the second whiff of ADHD. The first whiff is when my office manager, who has watched this boy destroy my waiting room, brings the family back and says to me, "Your next patient is ready" with the silent signal of bug eyes.

sleep study would show anything but normal sleep, but I wanted to be sure. They agreed, and we scheduled the sleep study.

~ ~ ~

If you are raising children, teaching children, treating children, or otherwise children-adjacent in some capacity, you are probably aware of attention deficit hyperactivity disorder. This disorder seemed to explode upon the scene and has affected not only countless boys and girls but has also become a common diagnosis in adults. While the disorder is clearly a multifaceted condition, it often has deep roots in the sleep health of children in whom it has been diagnosed.

A History of ADHD

Relatively speaking, ADHD is new by modern medical standards. Careful inspection of historical medical documents reveals cases and descriptions of the disorder dating back well over two hundred years. Formally described in the early 1900s, the disorder referred to children who were incapable of behaving themselves despite having the intellectual capacity to do so. Even with observational improvement in these children with stimulants, the disorder (referred to at the time as hyperkinetic impulse disorder) failed to reach widespread acceptance. Over the years, these behaviors were linked to the usual suspects: insufficient parenting (inadequate discipline, excessive discipline), poor diet, and a dearth of fresh air. By the 1980s with a new name, more treatment options available, and, more important, a rising knowledge and acceptance of the disorder, the incidence of attention deficit disorder sharply began to rise.

Although following the development of the disorder is fascinating, the changing view of its presumed underlying cause has a fascinating history all its own. Originally, the disorder was felt to be a "defect of moral control." Along the way to the modern understanding of the disorder, it has been attributed to "morbid alterations" of attention, a reaction to encephalitis, a direct outgrowth of experiencing early brain damage, and a fundamental underdevelopment of purpose. Of course, all these proved to be quite off the mark.*

What Is ADHD?

If we fast-forward to today, the current definition of ADHD tends to reflect a complicated mix of genetic tendencies, environmental influences, and other neurological factors that involve some disturbance of frontal lobe/executive functioning. The resultant disorder can greatly impact learning and the family and social interactions of the affected child.

This disorder is not rare. According to the recent work of developmental pediatrician Dr. Winnie Tso, the incidence of ADHD is somewhere between 5 and 15 percent of children. In Dr. Tso's research, and the studies of others, sleep amount and quality are important confounding variables and have to be taken into consideration when the diagnosis is made.

Symptoms of ADHD

On the surface, identifying the symptoms of ADHD appears simple. It's a child who is inattentive and has poor attention or concentration. While it is certainly true that inattentiveness is a central tenet of the condition, the outward manifestations in children are much more diverse and more difficult to pinpoint.

Generally, it is a child's behavior that immediately gets the wrong kind of attention from others. Often, this attention actively leads away from a diagnosis of ADHD and seems to be more of a manifestation of deficient behavior or an irritating personality. I'll admit it. My first thought when I walked into the exam room and saw Emory was, *Hey, Mom, do you think you could at least make your kid take off his shoes so I don't*

---

* Don't let that stop you from using "underdevelopment of purpose" in your own home. It's loads of fun.

"Dad, why did Coach take me out of the game? I had two really good at bats."

"Not sure, son, but guessing it was your underdevelopment of purpose in right field. What do you think?"

have to repaint my walls? His behavior was getting my attention and was clearly getting under my office manager's skin.*

Beyond these initial impressions, there are a host of symptoms both obvious and obscure that need to be evaluated. Often these kids are struggling. They are struggling to get into the flow of a household. They are constantly in the middle of mischief and conflict. At school, they are impulsive and argumentative. They can have trouble making friends, which leads to exclusions from sleepover events and birthday parties. Academic struggles can be present either because the content is difficult and requires concentration to master (acting out due to frustration or helplessness), or because content mastery is easy and thus becomes disengaging (acting inappropriately out of boredom).

Diagnosing ADHD

Diagnosis of ADHD is not easy because it can take time to adequately evaluate a child and screen for the many symptoms these children exhibit. The diagnosis of a child with ADHD takes time, medical expertise, and ideally lots of input as to the symptoms and behavior patterns of the child. While I do not want to go too far outside the scope of this book, I do think a look at the current diagnostic requirements can he enlightening.

The *Diagnostic and Statistical Manual of Mental Disorders*, fifth edition (*DSM-5*), diagnostic criteria for ADHD has changed over the years. In the past, there were ADD and ADHD, with the hyperactive condition having its own name. Currently both subtypes are referred to simply as ADHD, even though there remain two diagnostic requirements.

The inattention group requires that, of the following list, the child display six or more of the listed symptoms (five or more for adolescents seventeen years or older) for at least six months, and that the symptoms are inappropriate for the developmental level of the child.

---

* She refers to this as an individual "plucking her nerves." As a neurologist, I'm pretty sure that nerve plucking is impossible under most normal circumstances.

- Often fails to give close attention to details or makes careless mistakes in schoolwork, at work, or with other activities.

- Often has trouble holding attention on tasks or play activities.

- Often does not seem to listen when spoken to directly.

- Often does not follow through on instructions and fails to finish schoolwork, chores, or duties in the workplace (e.g., loses focus, sidetracked).

- Often has trouble organizing tasks and activities.

- Often avoids, dislikes, or is reluctant to do tasks that require mental effort over a long period of time (such as schoolwork or homework).

- Often loses things necessary for tasks and activities (e.g., school materials, pencils, books, tools, wallets, keys, paperwork, eyeglasses, mobile telephones).

- Is often easily distracted.

- Is often forgetful in daily activities.

For the hyperactivity and impulsivity group, it is the same thing. Six or more symptoms for kids up to age sixteen, five or more symptoms for seventeen years and older. Again, the symptoms need to be present for six months and be disruptive and inappropriate for the child's developmental level.

- Often fidgets with or taps hands or feet, or squirms in seat.

- Often leaves seat in situations when remaining seated is expected.

- Often runs about or climbs in situations where it is not appropriate (adolescents or adults may be limited to feeling restless).

- Often unable to play or take part in leisure activities quietly.

- Is often "on the go" acting as if "driven by a motor."

- Often talks excessively.

- Often blurts out an answer before a question has been completed.

- Often has trouble waiting their turn.

- Often interrupts or intrudes on others (e.g., butts into conversations or games).

In addition to the symptom checklist, *all* the following conditions must be met.

- Several inattentive or hyperactive-impulsive symptoms were present before age twelve years.

- Several symptoms are present in two or more settings (such as at home, school, or work; with friends or relatives; in other activities).

- There is clear evidence that the symptoms interfere with, or reduce the quality of, social, school, or work functioning.

- The symptoms are not better explained by another mental disorder (such as a mood disorder, anxiety disorder, dissociative disorder, or a personality disorder). The symptoms do not happen only during the course of schizophrenia or another psychotic disorder.

Just like everything else in neurology and psychiatry, it's not the most elegantly simple and straightforward process. While there are other tests, batteries, and assessments individuals can use to pin down the diagnosis,* this is the core of the diagnostic criteria.

Checking some boxes on a diagnostic criteria checklist is easy. Diag-

---

* I remember one specialist always asking if the kid liked to climb things. He said this was a common characteristic of kids with ADHD.

nosing ADHD properly is not. Notice anything missing from the diagnostic criteria mentioned? Hint: It is the overarching topic of this book. Yes, sleep!

To me this is a big deal because the interplay between sleep and ADHD is huge. Even though there are not additional criteria of . . .

The symptoms are not better explained by a sleep disorder.

. . . there should have been!*

Is this really a big deal? Absolutely. Sleep has always been a central behavioral component to ADHD. It is widely known that children with ADHD often have unique struggles and difficulties with sleep.

Sleep in Children with ADHD

There do appear to be specific changes in the sleep of children with ADHD. A 2004 study showed children with ADHD seemed to spend significantly more time in bed and exhibit more sleep cycles. Additionally, these youths seemed to spend more time in REM sleep compared to children without ADHD. They also displayed more movement during the night, particularly during light sleep. These movements often result in a more fragmented sleep. These are all aspects of ADHD in children that the sleep specialist reading your sleep study may not even be aware of!

Outside of the sleep study, there are also differences in the way children with ADHD sleep and manifest sleepiness. Children with ADHD can have significant difficulty with bedtimes, and these difficulties are often reported both by parents and the children themselves. Additionally, children with ADHD tend to sleep less and have more nocturnal awakenings than their similarly aged peers, a trait that typically emerges between the age of five and nine. Some studies have suggested a tendency for ADHD kids to be more phase-delayed (night owls). In a 2003 study, thirty boys between the ages of five and ten with ADHD were studied against age-matched boys without ADHD. In the study, the boys with ADHD were significantly sleepier despite no differences seen in the sleep studies of the two groups of boys. These studies (and many others) have led to a relatively clear understanding that children with ADHD do

* I wish people would ask me these things prior to going ahead without my opinion!

have unique and predictable changes in their sleep patterns. In the past, this relationship between ADHD and sleep disruption was mainly viewed in this direction:

ADHD → sleep difficulties in children

In other words, the sleep disturbances were an outgrowth of the ADHD; whatever the underlying brain process is that created ADHD also created observable sleep disturbances. Sleep disruption was a consequence of their loss of "moral control and morbid fidgetiness."

More recently, the opposite relationship has been more intensely explored, especially given the recent and rapid rise in ADHD diagnoses. Over time, doctors and researchers began wondering if the opposite relationship could be true:

Sleep difficulties → ADHD in children

The Rising Incidence of ADHD

Before we dive in, let's address the idea of rising ADHD diagnoses. Is it really rising? The short answer is yes, by virtually any metric. Results from published national survey data show not only a rise in diagnosis but a pretty remarkable one. Ignoring previous diagnostic categories and their specific criteria and only focusing on the *DSM-4* and *-5* definitions of ADHD, the diagnosis has risen from 6 percent of the population to 10 percent. Among scholars who study ADHD, there does not seem to be much dispute as to *whether* the diagnosis in children is on the rise. The real disagreement is about *why* it is rising.

Increased awareness on the part of parents, teachers, and health-care providers is most certainly a factor, as is a concurrent increased acceptance of the disorder as the stigma around it diminishes. The perception that the disorder creates an academic disadvantage clearly drives many to seek diagnosis and treatment in a college-competitive world. These theories tend to assume the number of kids who have ADHD is not changing, we are just getting better at finding them and accepting the diagnosis more readily.

The second theory is that the actual percentage of kids affected by ADHD is growing. In other words, there are actually more kids with the condition today than there were several decades ago. For those who subscribe to this theory, changes in sleep patterns and amounts are often central to the rising numbers.

It is impossible to discuss sleep in kids—particularly as it relates to ADHD diagnoses—without immediately invoking the scourge of technology.* There is data to back the relationship up. In a 2018 study, Adam Leventhal, PhD, a professor of preventative medicine at the University of Southern California, showed that the more engagement an adolescent had with technology, the more likely he was to display signs of attention disorders. Kids who reported little to no technology use displayed a 4.6 percent rate of attention deficit symptoms, versus a 10.5 percent rate in high users (fourteen high-frequency digital activities per day).

The keyword here is "relationship." Relationships between two things do not necessarily mean that one of those things *causes* the other. For example, I imagine that there is a relationship between Porsche hats and high-speed car crashes in the United States. In other words, if you examine the details surrounding these automobile accidents, you might find that there is a noticeable and alarming relationship between the crashes and the ownership of a Porsche hat. Are we to believe, then, that owning a Porsche hat might be putting the people in the hat owner's home in danger? No. The hat is not causing anything. It is simply a marker of high-performance car ownership, and individuals who actually possess cars capable of reaching two hundred miles per hour may be more likely to crash them.†

So how are we to interpret the ADHD and technology data? The obvious way would be that kids who interact with technology on a higher

---

* Also known as YouTube, TikTok, Snapchat, Xbox, PlayStation, *Fortnite, Call of Duty, Minecraft, Madden,* etc.

† I'm also pretty sure that wearing a Porsche hat indicates more concern about appearances while driving and less concern about speed limits and traffic laws.

basis are more likely to develop ADHD. This makes sense given the potential impact of technology and media consumption on a child's sleep.

There is another way to look at this data though. Perhaps the ADHD is already there, and the technology consumption is merely a marker for its presence. Perhaps the media interaction is a coping strategy or some other less obvious outgrowth of the condition.

Over the last five years, the balance seems to be tipping toward:

Sleep difficulties → ADHD in children

. . . and away from:

ADHD → Sleep difficulties in children

With nearly 80 percent of children with ADHD showing signs of circadian sleep disruption or other diagnosable sleep disorders, this change in thinking has led to calls for overhauling the core definition of ADHD.

So here is my assessment of the situation. Attention is the process of focusing your mental energy on something in your environment, monitoring information, and selectively responding to the items that matter in the moment while tuning out items that don't. This attention has a complicated relationship with sleep.

It turns out, impaired attention is a huge problem that results from sleep loss. In one study, subjects displayed three times as many lapses in attention if their sleep was restricted for a matter of just a few days. Restricted . . . not deprived! Think about this relationship as you examine how we typically treat attention problems. We use pharmacological stimulants. What else could a stimulant act to mask? That's right. Underlying sleepiness. So as the ADHD doctors are patting themselves on the back for figuring out what is wrong with your child, perhaps the stimulant therapy is not treating ADHD as much as it is covering up the real issue: excessive daytime sleepiness from some other cause. A 2006 study in Taiwan of 2,463 children ages six to fifteen showed that treating underlying sleep disorders was often enough to make the attention issues go away.

As someone who has followed the adolescent sleep and circadian research of pioneers like Mary Carskadon and James Maas, I strongly believe there is a causal relationship between sleep and ADHD. Further, I believe that sleep disruption creates deficits and disorders of attention that can get misdiagnosed in many situations. To me, there is really no other way to look at it.

With that position spelled out, I try to see the positives and negatives of both sides. What happens if I'm shown to be wrong in ten years? What if I'm right? Here's how I would break that down:

Option 1: I'm right—there is a relationship between sleep and disorders of attention.

If this is the case, we need to critically investigate a child's sleep because it can provide a diagnostic pathway and, more important, a treatment pathway for the uncovered sleep disorder as well as the resultant disorders of attention. If the treatment of the underlying sleep disorder (if found) results in attention improvement, we have just improved the life of a child and deepened our understanding of her disorder. If no sleep issue is found during the investigation, little to nothing is risked or lost, although the financial cost of the investigation should be considered.

Option 2: I'm wrong—there is no causal relationship between sleep and disorders of attention.

This option says that despite the available research on this topic, we take all diagnoses of ADHD at their face value, and we do not encourage the probing of the child's sleep history and quality. In doing so, while we may save a family money, time, and unnecessary interventions, we risk missing a potentially life-altering therapy for a child.

What it boils down to is simple—if I'm going to be wrong, I want to be wrong in the way that causes the least harm to my patients. A sleep study that leads to an intervention that does not improve a patient's attention is a much better outcome than blowing off a potential sleep disorder and its treatment that would have altered the medical course of that patient.

So, because I believe that sleep disorders often create attention problems, we always aggressively screen and look for sleep disorders in our patients with ADHD. I feel so strongly about the relationship that if someone asked my opinion, I would strongly recommend:

Do not let your child be diagnosed with ADHD without first having a sleep evaluation/sleep study.

How to Handle the ADHD Evaluation and Treatment

Despite one in five children potentially having an underlying sleep disorder contributing to or causing their ADHD (parent reports about sleep issues are often as high as 50 percent), subsequent sleep referrals to help determine if sleep issues are playing a role in the attention disorder are rarely made. This is where you may need to apply a little pressure. Typically, this is done through your child's doctor. I would like to say that this is a topic that will universally be discussed by pediatricians. It is not. Bring it up. Get a referral to a sleep specialist. Having the doctor directly order a sleep study is not good enough. There needs to be a sit-down meeting with the sleep specialist who will order and read the sleep study. Insist on this.

There is no risk involved in having a study, and if it illustrates absolutely perfect sleep, that itself is helpful information in the long run. If the study shows that there is a sleep disorder, fixing it could make a big difference in terms of your child's attention, school performance, mood, and many other aspects of her health and performance. When presented with that kind of compelling data, it is unlikely your pediatrician will argue about the referral. If he does, get a new pediatrician.

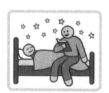

Treating Sleep Disorders and the Resulting Impact on ADHD

There are almost one hundred diagnosable sleep disorders that could be discovered with a sleep study. It is not necessary to dive into them all here. Suffice it to say that if the sleep study you fought for yields a diagnosed sleep disorder, treat it. It may very well improve or eliminate your child's ADHD issue. For example, in a 2012 study looking at children with ADHD diagnosed with restless legs syndrome (RLS), three out of seven children no longer met the criteria for ADHD once their RLS was effectively treated. In children diagnosed with mild obstructive sleep apnea syndrome, a tonsillectomy showed better improvement of ADHD symptoms than Ritalin.

Light Therapy

If the study is not indicative of a definitive sleep disorder, there is still work to do. Consider your child's circadian rhythm. While it has never been studied in children (and only twenty-nine adult patients were studied in the protocol), the application of bright light therapy in the morning was associated with subjective and objective ADHD improvements. Effects did seem to be enhanced during the fall and winter months because of the relative lack of light. To me, the use of light therapy in children who are generally phase delayed has no downside or risk. We have certainly seen improvements in our adolescent patients when light therapy is employed.

Sleep Program Intervention

Perhaps the most promising treatment for children with ADHD consists of interventional programs aimed at improving their sleep from a very early age. In a study of 244 children with ADHD, children and parents received two sessions of sleep intervention focused on improving the sleep of the children and educating caregivers. In the study, the children in the interventional group showed sustained improvement of ADHD symptoms and improved overall quality of life compared to control groups. The takeaway here is that acquiring quality information about sleep schedules, sleep environments, and sleep hygiene, when taught and implemented, can have a dramatic impact on ADHD symptoms.

Magnesium Supplementation

In a recent study of 116 children ages nine to twelve with a diagnosis of ADHD, up to 95 percent of those studied exhibited magnesium deficiencies. Magnesium supplementation acts to increase the brain's production of the neurotransmitter GABA, which has a calming and sleep-promoting effect on the nervous system.

Technology Intervention

Technology use in children with ADHD should be limited. While technology use is a big negative in my sleep book, there are limited studies that suggest video games can help to improve attention. The evidence is usually promoted by a technology company offering such promises as the fact that your daughter can play video games all day and concentrate perfectly well in doing so. The constant action, bright lights, and intense themes create an immediate rapid-fire stimulus/reward pattern that allows them to focus indefinitely. These devices and technology have been shown over time to hurt the attention and sleep of children. My recommendation is to limit its use, regardless of the form. For more information on this, see chapter 9.

Medication

While it is beyond the scope of this book to do a deep dive into the medications that are used to treat ADHD in children, these medications often fall under the category of psychostimulants. A list of common medications can be found in the appendix at the end of the book. Keep in mind the following slightly ironic twist: While ADHD medications can often be tremendously helpful for improving the attention and behavior of children, the relationship works in the opposite direction too. Disrupted sleep as well as sleep loss can also result from the treatment of ADHD once medications are introduced.

 Emory underwent an overnight sleep study and was able to make it through the entire procedure without leaving a single scuff mark on the sleep center walls. He fell asleep surprisingly quickly and slept well, according to both Emory and his mother, who stayed with him. A section of his study is shown here.

If you squint your eyes, you will notice what looks like a series of tiger stripes along the top half of the study. That is the pattern typically seen during a sleep study when an individual is chewing. The problem is, Emory is in bed, far away from a bowl of cereal when this is

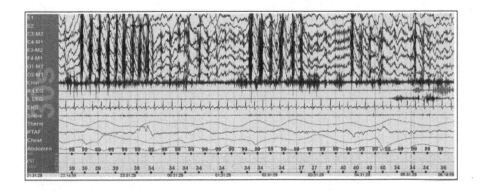

happening. That's because another cause of this pattern is a chewing movement made when an individual is having reflux disease at night, of which Emory was having a tremendous amount. This condition was not only responsible for his frequent awakenings during the night and his bad breath (remember the night breath?), but the disruption in his sleep was also responsible for his inattentiveness and poor behavior at school. This is not an unheard of finding, as a 2017 study in Iran found 55 percent of five- to twelve-year-old kids diagnosed with gastroesophageal reflux disease (GERD) in their study also met the diagnostic criteria for ADHD, compared to only 16 percent of the non-GERD children with ADHD. While we have seen this association in many sleep disorders, including sleep apnea, narcolepsy, periodic limb-movement disorder, nocturnal seizures, dust mite allergies, and cough-variant asthma, Emory was the first child we saw with ADHD symptoms from GERD. His symptoms improved dramatically once the GERD was addressed.

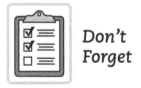

Don't Forget

1. Does your child exhibit signs of inattentiveness? Has this been brought to your attention by others?

2. Make sure a thorough evaluation is performed on your child, looking for other explanations of the behaviors in question.

3. Insist on an evaluation by a sleep specialist experienced with treating both children and individuals with attention issues. Strongly consider an overnight sleep study.

4. Depending on your child and views on medication, consider alternative treatments prior to medicating your child.

Narcolepsy

"Given How Much Your Child Sleeps in My Class, This C+ Is a Remarkable Achievement."

 It's not an uncommon occurrence to walk into my exam room to find a teenager soundly asleep on my exam table.

"Wake up, Sophie. The doctor is here."

Sophie woke up and smiled politely. She was clearly sleepy.

With considerable effort, Sophie was able to sit up on the bench and introduce herself. She was a student at the nearby university just getting started on her second year of studies and not doing well. Despite excellent grades in high school, her first-year college marks were a disappointment, and this year things were worse.

In my office, she was distraught that she had recently fallen asleep at a friend's house during a small party, and woke up to find pictures of herself on social media with soda cans and cats (seriously, you cannot make these stories up) stacked on top of her body. She was considering "taking some time off" after laboring through the second half of her first year when she was referred to my clinic by the college's student health services.

"I can't stay awake in class. I sleep all the time."

I nodded and asked, "How long has this been going on?"

Sophie mumbled, "A few months" as her mom simultaneously declared, "All of her life."

At this point, I asked Sophie if she would mind if her mom filled in some gaps. I told Sophie that if she disagreed with anything she said or wanted to add some details, she could at any time.

"Sophie," her mother began, "has always been sleepy. Initially, we thought she was a great sleeper. She always napped, always went to bed when we asked her to. Over time, the sleepiness seemed to become more extreme. Sleep became the only thing she was really interested in doing. She falls asleep in classes; she falls asleep as soon as she gets home. She sleeps away vacations and weekends."

"If this has been going on for so long, what made you seek help now?"

"Sophie was on the track team. One day during practice, she told the coach she had to go to the bathroom. Sophie never came back. After practice, the coach was cleaning up equipment after everyone had left. As he was leaving, he saw an equipment bag near some porta-potties adjacent to the track. As he approached them, he realized it wasn't a bag—it was Sophie, asleep on the grass."

Sophie grinned for the first time. "I totally did that."

With Sophie engaged, I asked a quick question. "Sophie, do you ever feel suddenly weak or paralyzed?"

Before Sophie could answer her mother interjected, "Oh God, the falling. That's a whole other thing."

"Actually, I don't think it is," I said.

~ ~ ~

Simply put, narcolepsy is a disorder of excessive sleepiness. Sleepiness that leaves parents thinking, *How can a human being who is not under some sort of enchantment sleep so much?* Sleepiness that has guidance counselors asking, "Is everything okay at home? Are you getting enough sleep?" Sleepiness that is so sudden and profound that it has pediatricians scratching their heads and incorrectly treating the symptom as seizures or depression. All the while, these sufferers of narcolepsy are constantly on a quest for sleep, regardless of the amount of sleep they receive. Kids with narcolepsy can literally get off the school bus, walk into their house, immediately fall asleep, and snooze until the following morning . . . and still fall asleep during second-period English class the following day.

Narcolepsy has other hidden aspects as well. The disorder features a collection of unusual symptoms that may not be as striking as the relentless slumber. Because of its effects on REM sleep, narcolepsy also comes with a host of signs related to dream-sleep dysregulation. Common indicators of the disorder include sleep paralysis, hallucinations upon falling asleep or upon awakening, and even experiencing the sudden paralysis of REM sleep while awake. This paralysis is termed "cataplexy," and it is often triggered by strong emotions like laughter or crying.

 The term "narcolepsy" was coined in 1880 by the French physician Jean-Baptiste-Édouard Gélineau to describe a wine merchant who was prone to sudden attacks of sleep, sometimes occurring two hundred times a day. This incredible disability and resultant loss of wine inventory almost certainly drove the merchant to seek help, as selling wine from a box would not be a thing for another eighty-five years. From the Greek words *narké*, meaning "stupor," and *lepsis*, meaning "attack or seizure," the word literally means an attack of unconsciousness.

Historically, excessive sleepiness and REM-related phenomenon like cataplexy were not considered part of the same malady. Over time, physicians linked the constant sleepiness with the accompanying signs to form the basis of our current diagnostic criteria.

What Is Narcolepsy?

Narcolepsy is a disorder of sleep regulation. The transition between sleep and wakefulness is so seamless in children. It is difficult to see with our eyes the neurological complexity involved when a child goes from being asleep in their bed to suddenly being awake and demanding French toast. A host of neurotransmitters are involved, many of which you have probably heard of: dopamine, histamine, GABA, acetylcholine. There is one particular chemical at the center of this condition that you may not be familiar with: hypocretin, also called orexin. (It has two names because two labs discovered it at the same time in 1998 and gave the chemical two different names. We will use hypocretin—no offense to the hardworking researchers in Texas).

In narcolepsy, individuals do not produce enough hypocretin, a chemical responsible for stabilizing wakefulness. Without the chemical, the ability to firmly remain awake is weakened, and the individual is susceptible to falling asleep without warning. Think about that for a minute; put yourself in a situation where you might feel sleepy: a long lecture . . . a church service . . . an endless dance recital. For most of us, we feel sleepiness begin to enter our brains. "Oh no! I need to do something or else I am going to fall asleep." We might get up, stretch our legs, grab a drink, or even pinch ourselves to create wakefulness. For many who struggle with narcolepsy, they never receive that warning. They literally walk into history class, excited to learn more about the Ottoman Empire, but soon find themselves waking up having never received any warning they were sleepy.

For years, narcolepsy was considered to be a genetic condition with the genotype HLA-DQB1*0602, commonly seen in patients who have narcolepsy, particularly with significant cataplexy. Recently, there is emerging evidence that narcolepsy is acquired via an autoimmune-mediated pathway. While the reasons for the immune system turning on itself are usually unclear, one specific example was seen in 2009 when a spike in narcolepsy incidence was seen following the Pandemrix H1N1 flu vaccine. While it has not been proven, there is some evidence to suggest that the immunization may have created an autoimmune narcolepsy in a small percentage of vaccine recipients.

Symptoms of Narcolepsy

Despite the often dramatic symptoms associated with narcolepsy, it is surprisingly difficult to spot. After being diagnosed, patients often remark, "I thought narcolepsy was when you suddenly fell over sleeping." This skewed perception is common not only in patients but also with health-care professionals as well, and it serves as a huge barrier for condition identification.

The symptoms of narcolepsy are simple:

- Excessive daytime sleepiness.

- Cataplexy: a partial or complete paralysis that is usually sudden in onset and short-lived.

- Unusual dreamlike hallucinations as the child falls asleep or wakes up.

- Sleep paralysis: an inability to move immediately upon conscious awakening.

- Fragmented nocturnal sleep.

Let's start at the top: 100 percent of patients with narcolepsy will have excessive daytime sleepiness (EDS). It may not be sleepiness that causes your child to fall over onto the ground asleep, but sleepiness should be a defining characteristic of your kid. One question I often ask parents or kids is, "If I asked your friends or relatives to describe you/your child, would 'sleepy' be a word they might use?" Another helpful question involves family nicknames or inside jokes. "Do people ever tease you about your sleepiness?"

This sleepiness is profound, constant, and unrelenting. Sleep helps some. Naps help a little, for a small period of time, but soon enough, your child is asleep again or complaining of being sleepy. Beyond sleepy, some kids develop a preoccupation with sleep that can border on obsessive at times. They literally wake up in the morning, stretch, and wonder when they can go back to bed. With stress and excitement acting to exacerbate sleepiness, it becomes very difficult for these kids to regulate their own wakefulness. For some, an anxiety develops over time to help combat the relentless drive for slumber. For others, they simply try to eat themselves awake, leading to the problems associated with overeating in narcolepsy.

Besides sleepiness, the remaining four symptoms, while very common, may not be present in every child, or they may present themselves at a later time. For example, in our clinic, we ask about cataplexy in different ways during every visit. It is remarkable how long it can take for it to either happen, or for the child or parent to recognize it.

To fully understand cataplexy and its relationship to narcolepsy, let's recall some things about sleep, particularly dream sleep, or rapid eye movement sleep (REM sleep). Roughly a quarter of our night is spent dreaming in REM sleep, with these REM periods broken up into distinct segments throughout the night, lasting anywhere from an average of ten minutes early in the night to about an hour later in the night.

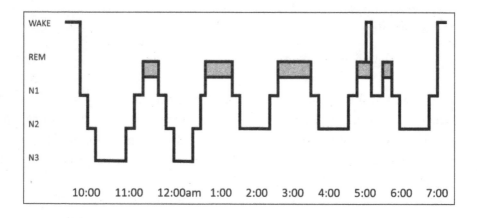

While important processes that involve memory function, concentration, attention, and even pain perception occur during REM sleep, perhaps the most interesting thing about REM sleep is the fact that we are all completely paralyzed while we dream. In a normal individual, this fact is rarely noticed because we are asleep and unconscious while all this paralysis neuroscience is happening. In children with narcolepsy, this paralysis can suddenly occur while the child is *still conscious*—actually awake and asleep at the same time. Imagine sitting in geometry class and being called upon to explain the triangle inequality theorem. Suddenly, all eyes are on you, and unfortunately, this is not something you reviewed the night before. While cataplexy can happen at any time, it is often triggered by episodes of high stress, and having everyone's eyes on you is not helping. As you prepare to formulate a verbal response, your jaw feels strange, and it is difficult to get your mouth to form words properly. Your neck goes limp and jerks backward like a sleeping father in church. Giggles begin to percolate around the classroom, ratcheting up the anxiety and worsening the weakness as the grip on your pencil relaxes involuntarily, and the pencil slips to the floor. Welcome to cataplexy.

In children, I have seen countless presentations of cataplexy, each unique:

- An inability to get up after being hit in dodgeball. Over time, the child realizes that he is not falling from the force of the ball hitting him but from the resultant cataplexy related to the stress of losing. This is not helped by the other kids laughing or yelling, "Faker . . . he's not hurt," as they believe him to be feigning an injury.

- A sudden loss of muscle tone during a school dance resulting in a boy's date almost having to hold him up during the dance. This resulted in chaperones immediately declaring a *Footloose*-esque PDA emergency, with the couple being unacceptably close to each other.

- A student being accused of public drunkenness because the cataplexy made her stagger. As the officer became more aggressive, her cataplexy worsened. In his report, he determined that this was "resisting arrest." (Note: this was a real case I was involved in as an expert witness.)

- A college student having a brief period of unconsciousness while on a ride at the town carnival (episodes can occur during fun experiences too).

- A child falling over in the hallway when a locker door was slammed, and the student thought it was a gunshot.

- A middle school student having unexplained episodes of slurred speech during class.

- A college student participating in a naked Slip 'N Slide event at a party ending up at the end of his slide in a naked ball, unable to move. Other attendees briefly thought there was a spinal injury involved.

Almost as quickly as it starts, the whole affair stops, and the child's muscles begin to work again. Taking the place of paralysis is often an overwhelming and uncontrollable urge to sleep. Children with narcolepsy often have incredible struggles with sleepiness throughout the day. Parents and children often tell stories of endlessly falling asleep in classes, and at sporting events, birthday parties, and even Taylor Swift concerts. My wife is a middle school English teacher who had a student with narcolepsy who had to move around the room to stay awake. If she insisted he sit down, he fell asleep within seconds. As a result, he often stood to complete work or take tests, just to keep from drifting off immediately.

Her student had been complaining of sleepiness to his primary care doctor for two years. But, as is common with many narcolepsy patients, neither the student nor his doctor may associate constant and ongoing sleepiness with the sudden and dramatic episode(s) of cataplexy. This may be true for a few reasons:

1. The child has never experienced cataplexy (it is thought that about 30 percent of narcolepsy patients will never experience cataplexy and only about 40 percent will experience it as an initial symptom either alone or with excessive sleepiness).

2. The child's cataplexy is so subtle that they don't notice it. The subtle and brief slurring of words with jaw weakness, a head bob, or a dropped cup may be shrugged off as incidental. Not all cataplexy is as dramatic as Sophie's. I call the dramatic cataplexy "Hollywood" cataplexy in my clinic, largely because every movie/television show that features narcolepsy always has dramatic (and comical) cataplexy, adding to the perception of the public that narcolepsy is rare, dramatic, and happens in hilarious ways during first dates and job interviews.* This is why it is so critical for

---

* Distorted depictions of narcolepsy are everywhere: comedy movies (*Spaceballs, Rat Race*), serious dramas (*My Own Private Idaho*), sitcoms (*Arrested Development, Frasier, Scrubs, The Simpsons*), TV dramas, and romantic comedies (*Ode to Joy*).

doctors of all types who take care of children to have at least a superficial understanding of the symptoms of narcolepsy, so they can recognize and diagnose it early.

3. The cataplexy is noticed, but not associated with the child's sleepiness. It is believed that the sleepiness is something else entirely.

The next symptom on the list, sleep paralysis, occurs when an individual awakens and cannot move for a short period of time. A child will become conscious, know he is in his room, but be completely unable to move or speak. While it can be terrifying for some, it generally only lasts for a minute or two (although a child who experiences it might feel like it lasted much longer and describe it as such). Sleep paralysis, while often seen in narcolepsy, is not a symptom exclusively seen in narcolepsy. Isolated events of sleep paralysis can also occur in individuals without narcolepsy, particularly when their sleep is chronically disturbed or they are getting an insufficient amount. My sixteen-year-old recently experienced it for the first time and was terrified. He said he saw a tall form coming toward

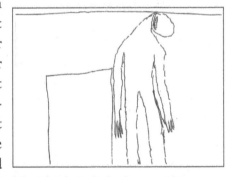

him, but could not move or scream. I had him draw it the next day.*

Hallucinations are another characteristic of narcolepsy. These hallucinations are commonly experienced as the child is entering into sleep (called hypnagogic hallucinations) or when they are waking up (hypnopompic hallucinations). These hallucinations are often rather mundane (the family cat seems to walk through the room, a conversation about remembering to pack gym clothes for the day, etc.). Often, these

---

* It's amazing how many people independently describe tall, shadowy figures, often who cannot fit in the room, when they have nocturnal hallucinations. It is known that figures are often distorted in dreams. Maybe this is the origin of Slenderman.

hallucinations are so routine that the child will have difficulty distinguishing conversations they had in real life from hallucinatory conversations ("I thought you told me you had packed my gym clothes for me . . . I could have sworn we talked about it!").

The final symptom, fragmented sleep, is a common feature of narcolepsy, and it stands at odds with the excessive complaints of sleepiness. If we consider the role hypocretin typically plays in stabilizing sleep and consolidating it, it is also serving the purpose to consolidate wakefulness. (If all the sleep is happening at night, there is no need for it to occur during the day.) In narcolepsy patients, it is not just their wakefulness being punctuated by periods of sleep during the day but also their sleep being punctuated by wakefulness during the night. This can become so pronounced in some kids that the entire nighttime picture seems almost more consistent with someone who can't sleep (and is therefore sleepy during the day naturally) than a child with a disorder of excessive sleepiness.

Diagnosing Narcolepsy

Diagnosing narcolepsy is a challenge. Unfortunately, early diagnosis of narcolepsy does not often occur. In fact, the average individual receives a diagnosis fifteen years after first reporting symptoms, with individual cases taking upward of sixty years to diagnose! In one review of 252 narcolepsy patients, 60 percent were misdiagnosed with conditions such as depression and insomnia before receiving a correct diagnosis.

In children specifically, the problem is worse, as narcolepsy is considered to be one of the most underrecognized and underdiagnosed serious pediatric medical conditions. The consequences of a failure to properly diagnose narcolepsy are far-reaching and may be complicated by the emergence of such seemingly unrelated conditions as poor school achievement, mood disturbances, obesity, and nocturnal bulimia. This association has been confirmed by a 2014 study of Finnish children, to name one.

If we do the math, it is easy to see why many patients struggle in school or eventually drop out, mistakenly feeling that they are not able to handle college or a stressful work environment. In other words, this particular missed diagnosis can often have a huge impact on the trajectory of a child's life and career. Take a look at these clues from a young woman's patient-intake form. She was later diagnosed with narcolepsy, seventeen years after her symptoms began in middle school.

Look at all the subtle clues pointing to narcolepsy:

- **"Some college":** She dropped out, likely because she simply could not stay awake in class.

- **Smoking:** Many narcolepsy patients accidentally find the stimulant effect of nicotine to be helpful in terms of staying awake.

- **No alcohol use:** Patients with narcolepsy feel tired all the time. Adding alcohol to the mix is usually the last thing they want to do, so alcohol use is minimal.

- **Caffeine use:** Caffeine is usually a crutch used by patients with narcolepsy to get through their day. (This patient had recently cut way back on caffeine because she was told by her primary care doctor that her excessive caffeine was the reason she was sleepy.)

- **Exercise:** When forced to choose between going to the gym or sleeping, sleep usually wins, so exercise is infrequent. In children, this often manifests as kids dropping sports in favor of coming home to rest before doing homework.

- **"Poor sleep quality":** One of the symptoms of narcolepsy is fragmented sleep.

- **Daytime sleepiness/fatigue:** Central to the condition.

- **Depression/anxiety:** Probably the most common misdiagnosis of patients with narcolepsy.

- **Weakness:** This is an exceptionally unusual symptom for an otherwise healthy young woman to indicate. This was her indication of cataplexy. The "numbness and tingling" was also related to how she felt during a cataplexy attack.

With it all in black and white, you might wonder why it is so difficult for these individuals to be properly diagnosed. In this example, the patient is slightly older, but similar clues exist for all kids. Despite the jarring nature of their symptoms, there are often two huge barriers that prevent health-care providers from getting it right:

1. They mistakenly think that the disorder is rare (so they are not looking for it, or if they find it, they think, no way it could be narcolepsy . . . it is too uncommon!).

2. They mistakenly think that all narcolepsy patients suddenly and dramatically fall over asleep while walking down the street (remember Hollywood cataplexy™?).

Narcolepsy is not rare, particularly when cast in the light of other disorders. Narcolepsy affects 1 in 2,000 people. Put into context:

- Cystic fibrosis is 1 in 3,000.

- Type 2 diabetes is 1 in 5,000.

- Parkinson's disease is 1 in 7,692.

In other words, you know someone with narcolepsy. In my world, I often meet pediatricians (or worse, pediatric sleep specialists) who make comments like, "We don't see a lot of narcolepsy where I practice." This is doctor speak for, "I don't know how to properly evaluate for and/or diagnose narcolepsy."

Because of these two barriers, doctors tend not to look for it (*It is rare!*), and when they see it, they miss it because they are looking for the wrong things. (*Ma'am, does your child suddenly fall over while walking down the street? No? I see, well, he's depressed.*) Fortunately, as time has passed, physicians are starting to think about narcolepsy and disorders of hypersomnia more, and even when they don't, parents are arming themselves with the right questions to get their kids to a sleep specialist's office.

You might think that once you've gotten your child to an office with "Board-Certified Sleep Specialist" on the door, you are home free. Not by a long shot. It has been estimated that fewer than 50 percent of sleep specialists are very comfortable either diagnosing or treating narcolepsy. Fifty percent! Can you imagine if 50 percent of obstetricians were not comfortable delivering babies? It is your job! So even after connecting the dots about your child's excessive sleepiness, there is a coin flip's chance that your sleep doctor won't know exactly how to evaluate your child in order to properly screen for and diagnose narcolepsy.

But wait, there's more. Even if your child is officially diagnosed with narcolepsy, many doctors are in the dark about effective treatment options. I routinely see patients who have been diagnosed with narcolepsy who are never offered the full complement of therapies. For some, it is because they are unaware or not up-to-date with current treatment options. For others, it is because they are not comfortable with therapies. In either case, kids and families suffer.

For better or for worse, the diagnosis of narcolepsy is largely clinical. In other words, it all hinges on the clinician's questions and the history she gathers from you and your child. These questions are essential to understand the nature and duration of your kid's symptoms. How long has he been falling asleep in class? What were his sleep patterns like growing up? Are there unusual aspects to the sleep? Is there a history of cataplexy? Are there other factors that could be contributing to the signs of sleepiness? As you can imagine, skill in this department and experience with the condition often go hand in hand.

The MSLT: The Narcolepsy Sleep Study

Once there is reason to think that your child might have narcolepsy, your doctor will probably discuss performing a sleep study. Unlike the sleep studies mentioned previously, this study will include an additional component: a multiple sleep latency test (MSLT). While the MSLT does not diagnose narcolepsy, its findings can go a long way to supporting a clinician's diagnosis.

So what is an MSLT? The MSLT will happen the day after the sleep study. Your child will undergo a typical sleep study at night and be awakened the following morning. After being awake for two hours (and having some breakfast), your child will be given the opportunity to take a nap. After the nap, your child will be asked to stay awake for another two hours. At the end of those two hours, it is nap time again. This pattern will repeat for the duration of the day. Five naps over ten hours, with the goal being to see how fast your child falls asleep during the day, and whether there are unusual expressions of REM sleep during the naps. The study helps confirm the diagnosis of narcolepsy if:

- the average time it takes your child to fall asleep is eight minutes or less, *and*

- there is evidence of two or more sleep-onset REM periods during the nap. (If your child went into REM sleep quickly during the overnight study, only one REM period during the daytime naps may be necessary.)

Note: Occasionally, it is acceptable to send a child home after only four naps. This can happen in one of two circumstances:

1. Your child is so sleepy that even a fifth nap in which there is no sleep (entered as a time of twenty minutes), averaged with the times of the other four naps, still results in an average sleep time (referred to as *mean sleep latency*) of less than eight minutes, *and* the child had already demonstrated REM sleep in at least two of the first four naps.*

---

* For the first time in my career, I had a patient undergo an MSLT, and her mean sleep latency was zero minutes. In other words, she fell asleep immediately in all four naps. Thinking about this patient, I suppose we could have ended her MSLT after three naps since even if naps four and five had been the maximum twenty minutes, this would have yielded a mean sleep latency of eight minutes, which meets the

2. Your child's sleep onset times from the first four naps are so prolonged that even a sleep onset time of zero minutes, averaged with the other four times, will result in a time longer than eight minutes, *and* the child has not demonstrated REM sleep in any of the first four naps, making it impossible to meet the criteria of at least two naps demonstrating REM.

It is important to understand that while this test can help to confirm the diagnosis of narcolepsy, the results, no matter what they are, *do not rule it out.* This is very important. In other words, if your child fell asleep in an average of two minutes but has only one period of REM sleep during a nap, it does *not* mean that your child does *not* have narcolepsy (sorry about the double negatives). Think of it this way—if a child was having multiple seizure-like episodes every day and a fifteen-minute EEG test done in a clinic was normal, that would not necessarily rule out epilepsy . . . even though the test did not support the diagnosis (it was normal). The test sure as hell does not mean the convulsing child is normal! Unfortunately, many sleep specialists do not understand this concept. In this example, a child fell asleep in an average of two minutes. TWO MINUTES! That is very abnormal! It is absolutely amazing how often I see kids with truly remarkable MSLT results that did not perfectly fit the criteria for narcolepsy (or did!), who were told that their studies were normal and they were sent on their way. It is not normal for a child to have wires taped and glued to their heads and, despite not being in their own bed, fall asleep in two minutes. If a physician wants to interpret an MSLT as "normal," that's her prerogative; that doctor still needs to provide an explanation for the child's exceptional sleepiness! This might involve repeating the sleep study and MSLT, or some other diagnostic test.

Sadly, the MSLT is a rather primitive test. It intrinsically has a false negative rate of about 30 percent . . . in other words, it will fail to

narcolepsy critera. Note: this patient had REM in her first three naps, so that criteria would have been met as well.

diagnose someone with narcolepsy about a third of the time. This is why you have to be diligent about making sure your sleep doctor understands the inherent pitfalls of diagnosing narcolepsy.* While there are genetic tests and spinal fluid tests for narcolepsy, they too are often not specific enough, not covered by medical insurance, or, more important, not recognized by insurance providers as evidence of the disease (despite the American Academy of Sleep Medicine stating otherwise).

Treating Narcolepsy

In the past, the landscape for treating narcolepsy was quite bleak. There were stimulants, some other kinds of stimulants, and that's about it. Recently, there have been several new and novel treatments approved by the FDA with potentially more on the horizon. For a complete description of these therapies, refer to the Narcolepsy section in the appendix at the end of this book.

I'm going to level with you. If you are sitting across from a doctor who has told you all these things and talked about all the drugs listed in the treatment appendix, I think you are home free. From this point forward, which therapies you choose for your child are decisions you will make as a team (i.e., parent-child-clinician). While I certainly have my own preferences and styles, I do not think that those belong in this book, as I

---

* Quick story. A failing student came to me with all the signs of narcolepsy and a sleep study that met the diagnostic criteria. To stay awake, she would often walk outside in the rain. After meeting with her and finding out her previous pediatric sleep specialist did not think she had narcolepsy, I wrote the doctor a one-line letter. *Dear ___, If this patient does not have narcolepsy, I'll eat my office chair piece by piece over a time period of no more than one month. Sincerely, Chris.*
The doctor called me upon receiving the letter and said, "I know . . . I didn't know what to do. She just seemed to have unrefreshing naps."

Hopefully this story illustrates just how even trained sleep doctors will sometimes run screaming from this diagnosis. By the way, this student has now graduated from college and is working on a graduate degree in biology.

truly believe that all these drugs potentially have their place in terms of narcolepsy therapy. I will leave you with a few thoughts on the matter of treatment:

1. You do not have to treat narcolepsy. Chances are, your child has been dealing with it for a long time. Maybe she's okay to continue living a sleepy life, or maybe some strategic naps every day might be enough to keep her functional. While I personally believe naps to be the equivalent of spitting on a raging house fire, they can work to some degree. Keep in mind, the goal here is to improve the quality of life in your child. Think about her being in a race with all the other boys and girls of the world. While everyone else gets to race on the smooth, paved surface of the track, your child is racing just off the track in six inches of mud. It is possible that despite the handicap, your child might be able to keep up, or even win the competition. If so, think how well they would do if you were able to get them running on the track with everyone else.

2. While narcolepsy patients are great at telling you they are better, they are awful at telling you they are normal. As a doctor who treats loads of narcolepsy, this is an ongoing challenge. It is easy for me to fall into the trap of self-congratulating when a patient tells me, "Thank you so much, Dr. Winter . . . you've given me my life back." It is very sobering when minutes later, I administer a sleepiness assessment to find that I have only succeeded in improving a tragically sleepy kid to a level of just awfully sleepy. In other words, their "improvement" is still your worst day. This is an essential concept when your child is telling his doctor that he's much better. "Much better" and "normal" can be miles apart. Don't settle for better.

3. A big part of not settling for better is the fact that your child may need more than one medication to feel her best. I believe, and I think that research would support me in saying, that most narcolepsy

patients are not going to be "fixed" with a single drug. Kids should have the opportunity to try many different drugs with the goal being to try to figure out (a) if a drug helps, and if so, (b) is it helping enough to make an overall difference either by itself or in combination with other narcolepsy meds. If your sleep doctor has your child on 10 milligrams of Ritalin, and he's trying to convince you that this therapy is fine when what you are seeing from your child tells you it is not, advocate for more aggressive therapy or seek a second opinion. In my experience, most well-treated narcolepsy patients look something like this:

- Sodium oxybate when they go to bed.

- Pitolisant when they wake up.

- Modafinil later in the morning and at lunch.

- Adderall available if they need it (soccer game, late-night studying).

4. Find a sleep specialist with whom you and your child feel comfortable communicating. The treatment of narcolepsy (or other truly rare disorders of excessive sleepiness, like Kleine Levin) is a long process that requires a fair amount of communication. How is a drug working? How can the clinician help your child's school or university understand the complexities of narcolepsy? Would your child do better with more testing time or more flexibility in terms of assignment due dates? Should your child be in a single dorm room? There needs to be complete comfort with your doctors as you tackle these issues.

Narcolepsy can feel like a daunting, scary diagnosis. As I like to tell my patients, the only thing scary about diagnosing narcolepsy is *not* diagnosing narcolepsy—in other words, living a life of unrelenting sleepiness and never knowing that it is a treatable condition. Unfortunately, I see this in older children (and adults) all the time. If someone had figured this out earlier, things may have changed drastically.

 Sophie returned after the sleep study and the following MSLT. I asked Sophie if she fell asleep in any of the naps. I knew the answer. I was curious to hear what she thought happened.

"I think I fell asleep in one of them. I'm not sure."

Her uncertainty was common. Many narcolepsy patients have very poor insight and perceptions of their own sleep.

"You slept in all the naps. It only took you an average of two minutes to fall asleep. You dreamed in three of the five naps."

"Yeah, I remember," she remarked, and laughed at the comment.*

Sophie easily met the criteria for narcolepsy, and we began treatment immediately. Fortunately, she had a remarkable response to the medications. Several years later, after her graduation, she sent me a long, handwritten letter of appreciation and her college transcript. On the transcript, she had annotated the various steps of her narcolepsy treatment. When she was diagnosed. When she initiated treatment with her first medication, modafinil. When she added a second medication, sodium oxybate. With each step in the process, you could clearly see her GPA improve from a 2.973 her first semester to an eventual 4.000 her final semester.

While she knew she could have done better in her first two years of college had she been diagnosed and treated earlier, she was nonetheless thrilled with the way she currently felt and was excited for the future (as opposed to when we met and she was feeling exhausted and considering taking some time off from college). Narcolepsy is not rare. It is in our schools and communities. Hopefully as more people learn about the disorder, we can shrink the time it takes for these kids to get the care and support they need to thrive.

* Again, the apparent conflict between an individual who remembers dreaming but did not think that they slept is the norm with narcolepsy patients.

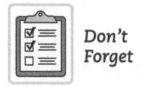 **Don't Forget**

1. Answer the following questions:

Does your child exhibit signs of excessive daytime sleepiness at home or at school? Is your child preoccupied with sleep or napping?

Does your child often ask to sleep or simply put himself to bed?

Is your child's sleep at night fragmented or unusually disturbed?

Has your child recently had an unexplained academic decline? Been diagnosed with ADHD?

Does your child exhibit periodic and brief episodes of slurred speech, weakness, head-bobbing, dropping things, or falling unexpectedly? Has your child been evaluated for potential seizures or fainting spells only to not be given any specific diagnosis?

2. If the answers to any of these questions are yes, it is important for you to consider the diagnosis of narcolepsy in your child and get professional help.

3. The diagnosis of narcolepsy has been called "the Great Pretender" because it can look like depression, anxiety, ADHD, and a host of other disorders of fatigue (thyroid, nutritional deficiencies, tick-borne illnesses, vitamin D deficiency). Make sure your doctor is considering this diagnosis, particularly if the treatments for the diagnosed condition seem ineffective.

8

Circadian Issues in Children and Teenagers

"Good Morning, Mom. What's for Dinner?"

Seeing two parents with a teenage child during a sleep doctor appointment means one of two things, and neither is good. The first reason may be that there has been a divorce, and neither wants to be blamed for anything medically wrong with their kid, so they have come to make sure they are present to defend themselves. The second reason is their child has something wrong with the timing of their sleep.* I just walked into the exam room, and there is a teenager with two parents. I quickly glance at the chart and see that both reside at the same address, and both are wearing wedding bands.

"Ferris, can you say hello to the doctor?" Dad prompts, and Ferris makes minimal eye contact.

---

* I really can't explain this phenomenon, I can only report it.

"He can't sleep. . . . He's up all hours of the night . . . always on his computer . . . that's the problem, I've been saying it for years," gripes Dad.

"The computer is the only thing that makes me sleep," snaps back the son.

Before we get to "We'll see how well you sleep when I throw that computer out of the window," I ask the question, "How many times have you been tardy this year?"

"A lot," his father says, while his wife says, "Forty-six" at the same time.

To this point, Ferris has said nothing to me. He is looking around for an exit. This visit clearly does not matter to him.

And why should it? Let me paint a picture of his life. He gets up anywhere between 10:00 a.m. to noon on school days and usually goes to class. He's tardy virtually every day. His parents try to wake him up, but after many unsuccessful attempts, they give up because they have to go to work themselves.

Ferris has little motivation for school, and he is quite behind from a work perspective. He has missed so much school that there is serious talk of homebound instruction. This discussion does not seem to concern Ferris whatsoever. Formerly a straight-A student, it is not a certainty that he will pass tenth grade.

"What do you do all night?"

"He's always on his computer, usually gaming or literally watching other people play games. War stuff . . . shooting people."

"It has nothing to do with war."

"Well, whatever it is, he plays it instead of going to sleep when he should."

"I've told you, I can't sleep, and the other doctor said it was because of my circadian rhythm, so it is not my fault."

Other doctor. Circadian rhythm. At this point, I know exactly what has happened prior to this visit. They have seen another sleep doctor, and that doctor ordered a sleep study. In the study, (1) the patient did not have sleep apnea, and (2) it took him a while to fall asleep. At the bottom of the report, three dreaded words appear: "circadian rhythm disorder." Under recommendations, there was nothing.

"I see here that you had a sleep study a few months ago."

"Yes, but the doctor said he didn't sleep."

Not true . . . his total sleep time was three hours twenty-eight minutes with his sleep onset at three fifteen a.m. and wake time almost seven a.m. I choose not to fight that battle at the moment.

"They said I have a circadian disorder."

"Okay," I answered, "and what was their plan to fix it?"

Blank stares and uncomfortable shifting in seats.

~ ~ ~

In the South where I grew up, "sleeping in" is not exactly a virtue. It was understood that being an early riser definitely put you in better favor with Jesus. I recall as a kid sleeping over at various friends' houses, how there were varied rules for sleeping in. In my house, my parents seemed to accept the fact that I was a night owl and liked to sleep in on the weekends. At other homes, most parents were not as lax about revelry. I learned quickly from whom to accept sleepover invites, and which kids I needed to persuade to accept an invitation to my abode.

If you ask any kid about sleep, you may get the impression that the amount of sleep matters less to them than the timing of their sleep. It is almost as if there is something more restorative about sleeping from 3:00 a.m. until noon, versus sleeping the same nine hours from 9:00 p.m. until 6:00 a.m. Why would that be? Isn't an hour of sleep just an hour of sleep?

It turns out that the answer is an emphatic *no*. The timing of sleep is an incredibly complex phenomenon that directly affects the quality and effectiveness. Understanding it can help you, as a parent, not only create the best setting for your child's sleep, but it also helps to understand and fix sleep issues that may arise as your child matures. Additionally, helping your child understand the effects of timing on sleep will better prepare her for adjusting and optimizing her sleep over her entire life.

What Is a Circadian Rhythm?

The idea of biological timing is relatively new when it comes to the process of sleep in children. The idea of timing as it relates to sleep in general is quite new as well.

In 1834, physician Robert Macnish speaks about sleep timing in his book *The Philosophy of Sleep.*

The character of the early riser is the very reverse of the sloven's. His countenance is ruddy, his eye joyous and serene, and his frame full of vigor and activity. His mind, also, is clear and unclouded, and free from that oppressive langour of which weighs like a nightmare upon the spirit of the sluggard. The man who rises betimes, is in the fair way of laying in both health and wealth; while he who dozes away his existence in unnecessary sleep, will acquire neither. On the contrary, he runs every chance of losing whatever portion of them he may yet be in possession of, and of sinking fast in the grade of society—a bankrupt both in person and in purse.

It is clear from his words that the individual who did not arise early to meet the day had a problem and was not going to enjoy the same kinds of success as the early riser. These biases were clearly reflected in Anna Steese Richardson's writing:

The child who has never known any habit except that of going to bed at six at night and waking up at six in the morning follows this course with little variation until he is old enough to learn from other children that one may sit up till all hours if one cries for it . . . and if he is allowed to do this he is started on one very bad habit, fretting and fuming until his wishes are granted.

These types of sleep problems have not gone away over the last century and a half, but in recent years, scientists have turned their focus on the timing of sleep to try to understand what is making teenagers like Ferris and his family "fret and fume."*

So far in this book, we have talked extensively about sleep need, and how the amount of sleep children require can vary from one child to another. We have touched upon the genetics of sleep need and how short sleepers and long sleepers (and everyone in between) have distinct genetic influences when it comes to the amount of sleep they require. That is all about sleep *duration*. What about sleep *timing*? It turns out that this is genetically influenced as well. To understand this, it will help to understand the concept of a *chronotype*.

Most people have heard of night owls. Maybe your kid is one. My daughter is. She loves staying up late and always has. Truth be told, so do I. What exactly is going on in a kid who simply seems to enjoy being awake more at night?

The concept of chronotype refers to the timing of that individual's circadian rhythm. Virtually everything our bodies do is governed by biological rhythms. If you want to see it in action, take your daughter's temperature every thirty minutes for the next few days. Chances are, you will see the data points form a remarkably consistent pattern that looks something like this:

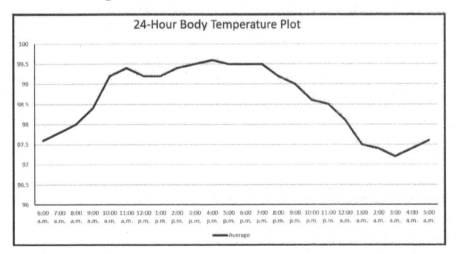

* It's like Anna Steese Richardson can see into the future!

What are we looking at here? This solid line shows an individual's body temperature fluctuations throughout a twenty-four-hour period, from 6:00 a.m. on the left, to 5:00 a.m. on the right, twenty-four hours later. Notice how our body temperature tends to peak around the late afternoon and suddenly drops to its lowest point (or nadir, one of my favorite scientific words), a few hours before we awaken.

What is so awesome about this graph is that day to day, the shape of it remains about the same. The pattern of our body temperature rises and falls in a predictable way, just like the tides, or a sunrise and sunset.

Now, what do you think would happen if we got a bunch of your daughter's friends together and measured their body temperatures over the same time period? Would their measurements show the same pattern? Not exactly. While the overall shape would be similar, you would probably get a graph that looked something like this:

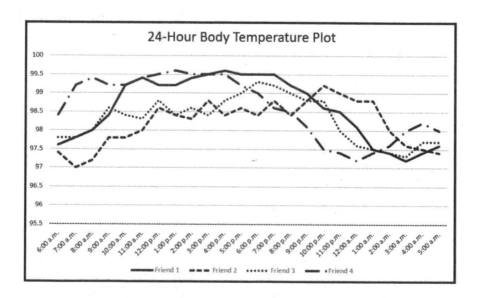

What you see in this graph is that each curve has roughly the same shape, but they seem to be shifted either toward the left or to the right of the original plot. The same overall biological pattern is happening, it's just rising and falling at slightly different times . . . some later, some earlier.*

Let me give you a glimpse into my home at night. In one corner (of the living room) we have my wife, who is covered in blankets and dozes on the couch. In the other corner, my sixteen-year-old son is dressed only in boxers and begging to stay awake a little longer, saying there is no way he will fall asleep if he goes to bed now, and that it is unfair to have to go to bed so early because nobody he knows at school is forced to do so. Thinking about the idea of chronotype and the temperature plot shown, what we see is the graph and chronotype come to life. Think of my wife as one of the tracings that drops early (friend 4). Her body temperature is the first to drop from the left, at around 8:00 p.m. Now look at my son's graph (friend 2), the farthest one on the right. If you look up from 10:00 p.m., his temperature curve is just peaking (hence the boxers and mega-wakefulness).

If I told you that body temperature drop was intimately tied to sleepiness, suddenly aspects of chronotype and the circadian rhythm begin to come into focus. Some of us are night owls. Night owls feel alive at night and sleepiness is not always conveniently found between 10:00 and 11:00 p.m. Night owls have what we call a *phase delayed chronotype*, and you can see that in the graph. Their curve drops later, or stated another way, their drop is delayed when compared to the baseline curve.

Conversely, some among us are morning types (sometimes called larks), and their circadian rhythm is advanced . . . a *phase advanced chronotype*.

What does this all mean? It simply means that the internal clock that we all have in our brain has different setting adjustments in different people. It is almost as if we were all given watches and allowed to set them with no standard. In other words, we all looked at the sky and made a guess. Some of us would be a bit late, others early. Regardless, our days would be the same . . . twenty-four hours. The difference would simply be that noon would happen at different times for different people.

* After being given a temporal thermometer, I actually plotted out my temperature over a twenty-four-hour period and it almost perfectly re-created this graph.

There is no watch inside our kids. What their brains do possess is a structure called the *suprachiasmatic nucleus*. This happens to be the central structure of timekeeping in our brains—it is the center of the circadian rhythm.

We have already explored one body function the circadian rhythm controls—body temperature. That's just the beginning of what falls under the regulation of a young person's circadian rhythm. Everything from digestion to hormone synthesis to athletic performance and blood cell production in the marrow of our bones is controlled by this rhythm. While it is true that even nasal congestion and which nasal passage is easier to breathe through has a circadian rhythm, there is one function that most people think of when it comes to the circadian rhythm—sleep.

Symptoms of Circadian Rhythm Disorders

Sleep and our circadian rhythm have become tied very closely together. We often think about circadian disruptions when it comes to teens and school start times. We even think about it as it pertains to kids sleeping in on the weekends or maybe getting up at 5:00 a.m. for a three-hour swim practice. Disorders that affect the circadian rhythm can have significant consequences regarding sleep, and kids can be particularly affected by these disorders. It is important to understand the unique functioning of the circadian rhythm in children and what happens when these rhythms are disrupted.

Before we begin, let's talk about children in general. I say "in general" because there are always exceptions to every rule. Typically, children tend to display a bit more of a circadian delay than older individuals, and in particular senior citizens. Because of this, children seem almost hardwired to want to stay up late and despise mornings. Conversely, their grandparents are ready for bed far earlier and are up before the sun.

In this chapter, I have chosen to focus most of the attention on children who have a tendency toward a circadian delay (night owls). Disorders around a delayed circadian rhythm are the most common circadian rhythm disorders seen in children.

A quick look at the different categories of circadian sleep disorders:

- Delayed sleep-wake phase disorder (these kids are night owls).

- Advanced sleep-wake phase disorder (these kids are early risers).

- Irregular sleep-wake phase disorder (these kids typically display erratic sleep patterns).

- Non-24 sleep-wake phase disorder (these kids would have sleep schedules not linked to a twenty-four-hour light cycle).*

- Shift-work sleep disorder (this would refer to sleep disruptions caused by unusual work schedules, uncommon in children, but could be seen in an older teenager who was working unusual hours).

- Jet lag sleep disorder (this would refer to sleep disruptions caused by travel over multiple time zones).

With a focus toward children, I'm not going to engage in a lengthy dialogue about jet lag. If you have an eight-year-old who is traveling around the world because she is an international YouTube celebrity: (1) congrats, I think, and (2) there are plenty of adult resources about combating jet lag.

So back to our little night owls. For the most part, all of this would be of minor consequence were it not for schools. We have already given our schools and their early start times a hard time in chapter 5. Now let's consider the start time from a kid's circadian perspective.

We previously listed a number of body systems that rely on the circadian rhythm for timing. Biologist and cofounder of the field of chronobiology Jürgen Aschoff once wrote, "Whether we measure, hour by hour, the number of dividing cells in any tissue, the volume of urine excreted, the reaction to a drug, or the accuracy and the speed with

---

* This is almost entirely a disorder of individuals who are completely without sight because they lack the typical light cues. It could be argued that this is also seen if you live in places like Northern Canada/Alaska, etc., where inhabitants often experience prolonged periods of darkness.

which arithmetical problems are solved, we usually find that there is a maximum value at one time of day and a minimum value at another." Intellectual and cognitive performance is no different. Just like we can measure body temperature's ebb and flow throughout a twenty-four-hour period, so too can we measure a sixth grader's scholastic performance. Care to hazard a guess as to when that process reaches its peak? At what time is your daughter most likely to crush her spelling quiz and actually spell "restaurant" and "acquiesce"? Four p.m. That's right! She will academically peak about an hour after the average school day ends!

This example provides a sense of how the symptoms of circadian disorders often manifest themselves. In general, these symptoms are related to timing mismatches. In other words, nobody would be surprised if your daughter's performance on that spelling test was subpar if she was awakened at 3:00 a.m. to take it. She's taking a test in the middle of the night! We all know that 3:00 a.m. is not an ideal time to be examined. Furthermore, we would all assume that 11:00 p.m., while better, would not be ideal as well. In broad strokes, we understand that there are generally better times and less ideal times to take the test.

So just like we measured our body temperature over thirty minutes throughout the day, imagine plotting out "spelling ability" over twenty-four hours. We would see roughly the same curve emerge. Some times are generally better for remembering "*i* before *e* except after *c*," and some are worse. Moving past temperature and spelling, if we kept plotting all the things our bodies and minds do in a day, we would create one similarly shaped plot after another, each with a twenty-four-hour rise and fall. That's what the term circadian actually means—"about a day" or about a twenty-four-hour period.

In this example, it is easy to see how academic performance in a child could be a big clue that there is a circadian rhythm disorder. In fact, having some sort of academic or social struggle is central to the diagnosis. The other clue, as demonstrated by Ferris, is extreme difficulty falling asleep and waking up. Once again, the mechanism for doing so works, it's just out of sync with the "right" times for it to work. The internal clock is mismatched with the homeroom clock, so to speak. If the school contacted Ferris and said, "Just come when you can. We'll get started as soon as you arrive," there would be less of a problem.

These are the more obvious outward signs of the disorder. Less obvious signs point to other biological rhythms more difficult to observe. Changes in mood, energy, motivation, and even appetite are apparent. Imagine how hungry you would be for a hamburger at 2:00 a.m.! What food options are available to a teenager who feels ready for dinner at midnight?

Delayed sleep-wake phase disorder (DSWPD) is not rare. It affects 7 to 16 percent of children and is particularly prevalent in the teenage population. Of the children who present with "insomnia" in my clinic, a high proportion have this disorder as either the primary cause or a secondary contributor. Genetics play a big role, with 40 percent of affected children having an affected family member. Moreover, this disorder carries with it a much higher risk of concurrent psychological disorders like anxiety, depression, and even ADHD!

Determining Your Child's Chronotype

As a parent, you probably have a pretty good feel for the chronotype of your children. It pays to consider your child's chronotype because just like being informed about the amount of sleep your child needs, having a feel for the ideal timing can guide you in your decision-making as well.

Given the highly genetic tendencies of chronotype and circadian rhythm disorders, step number one is a look at the family tree. If Dad is a night owl and finds it hard to get into bed before midnight, guess what? Daddy's little boy might have a bit of the night owl in him too.

With so much at stake, is there a way to more precisely determine the chronotype of our children? If you want to be scientific about the process, and your child is old enough to answer some simple questions, there are actually questionnaires they can answer. The most commonly used is the Horne and Östberg questionnaire, sometimes referred to as the Morningness-Eveningness Questionnaire (MEQ). The downside with this tool is that it was written for adults, although researchers have modified to be used in children. Another simpler assessment uses the midpoint of the sleep period on an unscheduled or "free day" as the chronotype determinant. In other words, what is the time midpoint between when your child goes to bed and when he wakes up on a weekend or otherwise school- / schedule-free night?

To me, the most useful measurement tool for kids is the Children's Chronotype Questionnaire (CCTQ). The CCTQ was developed in 2009 by Dr. Oskar Jenni, director of the Child Development Center in Zurich, Switzerland. In this twenty-seven-question survey, a parent answers questions probing the child's sleep tendencies both on "scheduled days" and "free days." When does she prefer to go to bed? When does she prefer to wake up? How does she wake up? Once all the questions are answered, the answers are assigned a point value. Simply add up the numbers and voilà: you have a morningness-eveningness quotient ranging from 10 (extreme morningness) to 49 (extreme eveningness). They further subdivided their subjects as follows:

morning types 10–23
intermediate types 24–32
evening types 33–49

This number, or any chronotype assessment, is a powerful bit of knowledge to have. Not only does it allow you to see where your child is on the chronotype spectrum, but it is a very helpful piece of intel to have when dealing with schools, doctors, or other individuals as it relates to your child. Does having a very high (or very low) score necessarily indicate that there is a problem right now? No. A child can score in the forties, and while it clearly shows a tendency toward having a delayed circadian rhythm, it does not mean he has delayed sleep phase disorder. But even in a child who seems to be doing well, the number might be suggestive that he is at risk in the future. For children whom you suspect have circadian rhythm disorders, this number can be very helpful in terms of having more objective findings to give to a school or medical professional. Fair warning. You may need to explain what a chronotype is to that individual!

One final note about a chronotype assessment. It's generally not a static number. It can change over time, in positive ways and negative ways. Just because a mild night owl is doing okay now does not mean that things can't worsen in a year. Conversely, by employing some treatment strategies listed later in this chapter, you might find that a child's more extreme night tendencies lessen over time, and the chronotype assessment can be a great way to measure that treatment's success.

How to Address Circadian Rhythm Disorders

Circadian rhythm disorders are often misunderstood, even by diagnosing physicians. In my experience, it often seems like the label is given to a child, and that's it. No treatment, just a shrug as if to say, *Your kid likes to stay up late. Nothing we can do about it.* Kids and their families leave as if they have been diagnosed with some terminal illness. With one patient, the sleep doctor had endorsed homebound instruction, almost as if that was the best that could be done.

Nonsense. There are many things that can be done about a circadian rhythm disorder. There is one little catch in terms of treatment success, and it can often be wrapped up in a very simple question.

Is the patient interested in fixing the problem?

The success or failure of treating circadian rhythm disorders often boils down to one simple factor—motivation. If the idea of homebound instruction and constant access to video games becomes the motivation, treatment is going to be challenging. One question I often pose to the family of an older child is this: "If your house caught on fire, would your child perish in the blaze, or could he save himself?" Despite the morbid nature of the inquiry, it gets to the heart of the issue—motivation. Can they get up to go to school? No. That's why the child is here. Can they get up for their travel baseball game, or other fun activities? Often the answer is yes.

I always make a joke at this point. "If I cannot fix a child, there is an army drill sergeant who can . . . typically within a week." When I say that, I'm sending two messages. The first message is to the kid. There are people out there who are a bit more motivated to wake you up in the morning, and they will go to great lengths to do so. The other message is to the parents. You need to be more like these people.*

* While my son is not in the army, he is at the United States Naval Academy. He is not aware of any circadian rhythm disorder that the United States military is unable to "remediate."

I'm not usually one for assigning blame, but let's assign blame. Who is responsible for a child waking up in the morning? If you answered "the child," I'll accept that. It is her future on the line if she does not make it to school, do well, and get grades good enough to secure a college invite. She should be motivated to get up. Ferris is, however, a kid, so I think his parents do shoulder a portion of the responsibility. While I certainly understand how important it is to work, and be on time for work, it is also important that their son not miss school.

Remember when I told you that I was a night owl? Well, that is not a new thing. I have always been drawn to being awake at night. I still like being awake at night, but life, work, and family act to temper those tendencies. When I was in school, there was another factor that dampened my night owl ways. His name was Bill Winter. He's my father. He played linebacker at Marshall University back when helmets were made out of shoe leather, I think.

I think of him often when I see kids like Ferris.

"We go into his room to wake him up, but he says for us to get out, and that he's too tired to go to school. He says he was up too late and that now he has to sleep."

I think of my father because I imagine myself as a fifteen-year-old, laying that line on him in the morning as he is getting ready for work.

"Get out, Dad, I'm too tired! I need—"

At this point I imagine his gentle hands lovingly scooping me up from my bed. I'm wearing a pair of boxers. I imagine him putting me into his driver's education car and rolling up to the front doors of Glenvar High School. I picture the scene in the movie where the wounded mobster gets dropped at the doors of the emergency room before the car tears off into the night. Suffice it to say, my father, like everyone else, has had struggles in his life. Getting his children up and to school was not one of them.

Having said this, if a child is not actively engaged in the solution of this problem, it can be much more difficult, particularly when said child is bigger than you are.

At what point does a family decide that a delayed sleep tendency has crossed over into a true disorder, requiring a diagnosis of DSWPD? In general, the following criteria are used:

- Is your child's sleep more than two hours delayed from what would be considered normal for that age group?

- Has this been a problem for more than three months?

- Is the delay causing significant social- or school-related issues?

As with most disorders in this book, the "two hours" and "three months" criteria are just guides rather than a hard-and-fast rule that must be met before you seek help. A student's academic year can be ruined in a month or two, so no need to wait before taking action.

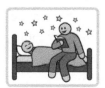 Step one of dealing with a circadian rhythm disorder is that you have to be tough . . . kind, but tough. It is well known that some kids with this disorder have little interest in doing the work necessary to fix it. They expertly play upon the sense of sympathy that parents have for their children. When a parent hears their teen walking around in his room all night, it is natural to feel for him. Entering his bedroom early in the morning, it does not feel kind, compassionate, or frankly healthy to awaken him for school after only a minuscule amount of sleep. It is, however, a must. Remember earlier in the book when I talked about consistent wake times being very important?

Think of it this way. You are in a battle for his soul. It is you against his mutinous brain; a brain that has developed a certain taste for leisurely noon awakenings. It is up to you to send a message to your child's brain that no matter what it decides to do in regards to sleep at night, wake time is every day at 7:00 a.m. to get ready for school.* Expect resistance. I have heard stories of children saying absolutely awful things to their parents. Like a scene right out of *The Exorcist*, your child's head may turn 360 degrees, and profoundly hurtful things might be said.† You must be

---

* Weekends too!

† "I cast you out of bed!"

strong. That kid needs to be out of that bed when the alarm goes off. Period.

The first step in treatment is to stabilize the schedule. It's no different than a trauma situation. Get a hand over that laceration and stop the bleeding. Kids with DSWPD tend to start small and gradually up the disconnect between "ideal time" and "their time." Hopefully, you are reading this and thinking, "Thank goodness my sweet little tots don't have DSWPD." By being armed with this education, you may notice your kid start to push sleep later and later on the weekends as he grows up. Maybe he really begins staying up late on vacations and sleeping in. Being aware of the disorder and how the process builds can help parents address the problem before it gets out of hand. Here's a pro tip my mother-in-law used on my wife. Vacuum the house, including the kids' bedrooms, at 7:00 a.m. every morning. My wife's internal clock is set to wake up early, and she swears it is because she was not allowed to sleep in as a kid. She may be right!

Once the schedule has been stabilized, it's time to work on improving the misalignment. If you can arrange it so your child has a nine-to-five job and twin babies, I've found that tends to fix the problem quickly. Otherwise, the most common method is to gradually advance (make earlier) the bedtime and wake time by fifteen minutes each one to two days, with emphasis primarily on the wake time. It cannot budge, nor can the affected child be allowed to nap at all prior to bedtime.

For some extreme cases, or if your child has been going to bed much closer to his necessary wake time, sequential *delays* in the schedule can be considered. In other words, work forward, delaying the schedule. Working forward and having your kid stay up progressively later (what he wants to do anyway) allows you to move faster. Keep delaying the bedtime and wake time by two to three hours every night or so until you work around the clock and arrive at the desired bedtime. For example, a child with a 4:00 a.m. bedtime would go to bed at 6:00 a.m., 8:00 a.m., 10:00 a.m., 12:00 p.m., 2:00 p.m., 4:00 p.m., 6:00 p.m., 8:00 p.m., and finally arrive at a more desirable bedtime of 10:00 p.m. nine days later. Obviously a 2:00 p.m. bedtime is not easily paired with school attendance, so this method's temporarily unusual schedule is a drawback. I would also caution against teens driving during this period of realignment.

Keeping a graph or chart about bedtime and wake time can be helpful in not only addressing and fixing the problem but maybe, more importantly, it allows the parents and child to see the progress. I like to use a simple "color in the block" schedule on graph paper.

Once you have arrived at the desired schedule, the work of maintaining the schedule really begins. It is of paramount importance that everyone is working to make sure he is awake at all times he's supposed to be. Check on him doing his homework. Make sure he's not asleep with his head on a textbook. Again, you are working to cut off all other access to sleep outside of the upcoming night.

Beyond the ruthless nap embargo, there is more work to be done. We previously emphasized the changes that happen in the brains of children when they wake up. We want those changes in this situation to be even more amplified. The use of light, or phototherapy, can help manipulate circadian patterns, and stabilize sleep cycles. Despite its long time use for mood disturbances (e.g., seasonal affective disorder), its use to influence sleep patterns is much more recent. When your child is awakened in the morning, there needs to be light everywhere—right away. If it happens to be a season in which it is dark when he awakens, that needs to be remedied. Consider purchasing a light box and exposing him to it when he awakens. There are alarms that utilize a gradual increase of light in the morning. Like a picturesque sunrise on your son's bedside table, these alarms expose your child to a brightening light source to help him wake up. Once awake, particularly on the weekends, do not let your child retreat to the dark basement dungeon and begin watching Netflix.

Breakfast is not optional. Remember that your child is, as far as his brain is concerned, waking up early . . . very early . . . maybe hours and hours earlier than what it is used to. Appetite may not be particularly robust. Think about how you would feel if you were awakened at 3:00 a.m. and presented with a poached egg and a side of bacon. Work with your child. Even consuming a couple of Saltines will send the appropriate message to his brain that this is morning, and it is time to eat. In an effort to get that light exposure up, consider serving the orange juice and Saltine outside in full sunlight!

Get your child active as soon as possible when the alarm goes off. Simply moving from an inactive heap on their bed to an inactive heap on a couch is not acceptable. Get outside. Walk the dog. Ride a bike or shoot some hoops. If your child is small, throw him in a jog stroller and hit the pavement. Exercise, first thing in the morning may be the singularly best thing for sleep at night!*

A cooler bedroom (around 65°F) is best for sleeping, so get the temperature down prior to bedtime. When sleeping is over, it is a good idea to warm the child's body up. If you recall from those temperature curves, when a child is on a good schedule, her body's temperature begins to rise a few hours before getting up. We want to continue that temperature trend in her after she awakens. Exercise, as mentioned, can accomplish this task, as can moving to a warmer part of the house, bumping up the thermostat a bit, or going outside when appropriate. There are devices like the Ooler that can not only cool or warm a bed but can actually be set on a timer to begin to slowly warm the bed prior to your child's wake time in an effort to make waking easier!

This plan should sound familiar. Thinking back to the earlier chapters in this book, it's not difficult to see the connections between establishing heathy circadian (and sleep) timing when a child is young. A baby's brain is very plastic and easily molded. Early establishment of good habits can make the treatment of circadian issues when a child is older much easier.

At this point there are no FDA-approved medications to treat pediatric circadian rhythm disorders. Despite this, some medications may be considered by your child's sleep specialist.

Keep in mind, if your child is slow to adopt these changes, or refuses to do so altogether (e.g., she refuses to stop napping or will not exercise outside), there may be more than just a simple circadian disorder at play. Conditions like chronic fatigue, mononucleosis, tick-borne illnesses, and other poorly defined conditions can impact treatment trajectory and success.

---

* Remember my military example? Think about how their days begin every day. PT (physical training), outside, first thing in the morning. It is the absolute best thing for circadian realignment.

Ferris's parents got to work. The visit to my office unleashed the Kraken on the poor boy. Between Mom's ferocious investigation of the chronotype determination (surprisingly, just a 31 on the CCTQ) and embracing the schedule, as well as Dad's new license to wake Ferris up via any means necessary, I'm not sure Ferris knew what hit him. There was a general agreement that it was going to be easier for Ferris to progressively delay his schedule rather than to try to slowly advance it. What was a few more days of missed school at this point?

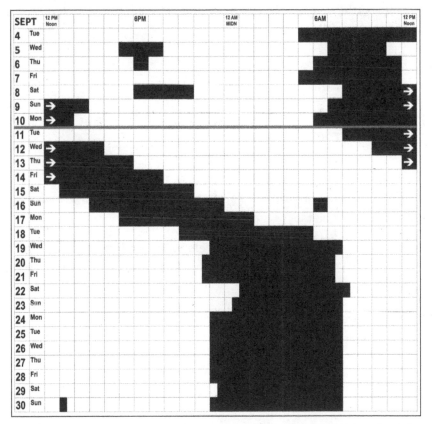

This chart represents Ferris's sleep over the the 27 days of his schedule adjustment. Each horizontal row indicates a day, with black boxes indicating hours slept.

Within a few weeks, Ferris was on track and doing "better than expected." His mood was not great. He was edgy and irritable but "willingly participating." His mother elaborated, "Ferris isn't dumb. He knows the next two years of school are important, and he wants to do well."

The intervention began after the tenth.* Starting Monday night, bedtimes were gradually shifted later, typically by two hours. While he was literally homebound the first week (his father did not work outside the home and was able to keep an eye on him), the process worked quickly and efficiently. Ferris was able to keep the schedule and over time grew to like it and the way he felt on it. He did go to college and, at last report, wants to be a teacher.

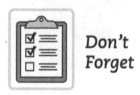 **Don't Forget**

1. Sleep timing is as important as sleep amount and often is the basis of a child's sleep problem.

2. Most children are predisposed to develop issues related to delays in their circadian rhythms, making it hard to go to sleep on time and get up regularly in the morning.

3. The disorders are common and can negatively impact school achievement and social interactions.

4. They take some work and participation to fix.

* Ferris "needed a week to prepare."

Technology and Children

"There Will Be No Television Until You Finish That Homework on Your iPad!"

 Remember Mike Teavee from *Charlie and the Chocolate Factory*? Mike was the fourth golden ticket winner in the book. He didn't like chocolate but loved television. He was obsessed with it.

I've met the real Mike Teavee, except his name wasn't Mike. It was Tiffany.

Tiffany is a seventeen-year-old who showed up at my office with her father, who was deeply concerned by her lifestyle, particularly her electronics use and gaming and their effects on her sleep.

The problem was not new.

Tiffany was introduced to *Minecraft* by her older brother when she was twelve. While his interest in *Minecraft* and video games in general waned over time, Tiffany's grew. Dad is standing in my office, arms crossed, and the first thing out of his mouth is this combination greeting to me and backhanded insult to his daughter. It goes something like, "Dr. Winter, thanks for seeing Tiffany. I'm not sure her problem is something you can fix unless you can tell my daughter how difficult it is to pay a mortgage and keep food on the table . . . unless you know of anybody hiring block builders, am I right, Doc?" He chuckles proudly.

Not knowing much about video games, I innocently ask, "Isn't *Minecraft* a game for little kids? Isn't it like LEGOs?"

She laughs at my complete ignorance. "The average player is twenty-four years old. And it is so much more than LEGOs. It's like my own world. It's an endless sandbox. You can do whatever you want."

"Could you do your homework in the *Minecraft*?" quips Dad.

"Why do you always call it *the Minecraft*? It's just *Minecraft*. One word." Tiffany huffs, irritated by the conversation about the game and probably the fact that she is here and not playing it.

I smile politely and look directly at Tiffany when I ask, "How can I help you?" It is really important to immediately gauge a child's interest. Are they in my office because they want to be, or are they there because someone else is forcing them to go? This time, there's no eye contact and no reply, which actually is a very loud and clear reply.

"The kid can't sleep, so she's up all night wasting her time on that computer. I vote we throw the whole thing into a lake: problem solved." I love this certain type of dad. His posture tells me he clearly does not want to be here and would much rather be back at the office. I'm guessing his wife insisted on the visit. The situation leads Dad to try to explain and treat the problem in one to two sentences with the solution generally involving something being thrown out a window or into a body of water.

"It is not a waste of time. People pay to watch me play." We are but a few minutes into the visit and already we have a child who has technology in her room and a raging sleep disturbance. Instead of sleeping she is not only playing video games on her computer but livestreaming said games so that other kids (I hope not adults) can disrupt their own sleep by Venmo-ing Tiffany money so that they can stay up to watch her play all night. Tough choice: video games and money versus homework and sleep.

Tiffany mutters, "It is more money than you make, Dad, and I can't sleep without the computer in my bed."

"How much are you sleeping, Tiffany?" I ask.

Looking at me for the first time, Tiffany says, "I don't sleep much. Games help me sleep though. They relax me."

"How much sleep are you getting?"

"Three to four hours a night during the week, and more on the weekend when I sleep in."

"I don't think that's enough sleep."

"It's enough for me."

~ ~ ~

In 1972, the surgeon general of the United States Jesse Steinfeld headed an effort to evaluate the dangers of television on the youth of America. Did watching television lead to more violent behavior? The results of the study, titled *Surgeon General's Study of Television and Social Behavior*, largely concluded that television was not making the majority of our youth violent and dangerous individuals, but that maybe some pockets of youth were more susceptible.

And in some way or another, the fight has continued ever since. Unfortunately, children today have more forms of electronic media at their fingertips than a single television in the family room. In fact, there are more advanced electronics and computing power in your son's iPhone than John Glenn had in his Mercury capsule when he orbited Earth.* If you were to ask me what the single biggest obstacle is for kids to achieve good sleep, it would be entertainment technology.†

On a personal note, I have three children. I think they are smart,

---

* It's interesting to think about the video game *Space Shuttle Simulator* and how this very complicated simulator probably uses far more sophisticated computing power and is more difficult to master than Glenn's relatively simple craft.

† In her 1913 writings on television, smartphones, and widespread gaming, Anna Steese Richardson famously said, "I have no idea what you are talking about."

capable, and kind individuals who, for the most part, are not terribly difficult to parent and absolutely cause my belief in the nature/nurture debate to swing more toward the former. That said, if you were to ask me what the single biggest challenge for me has been in terms of their upbringing, that's easy: their [insert favorite expletive] phones and computers.

Entire well-researched books have been written on this subject, so I do not intend to rehash all the dangers these devices pose to kids in this book. What I want to do is to stick to what I know—sleep and brains— and make some hopefully helpful connections to what you may be dealing with in your life.

Kids arrive in my clinic slouched over their phones, heads down, making no eye contact as they roam virtual worlds, executing soldiers and rummaging through their bloodied corpses for money and equipment. The parent is always there, smiling apologetically, indicating that despite their son's absent manners, he's actually a great kid and they, in turn, are a good parent.

As you can imagine, there are many things to deal with when it comes to a child's sleep, and the role electronics play in getting a healthy period of rest is a big one. While these stories often point a very strong accusatory finger at the cell phone and laptop, a good sleep specialist never rules out the presence of an underlying sleep disturbance based upon an initial visit and some stories about *Minecraft*. I have been fooled by plenty of "Tiffanys" who turned out to have raging sleep apnea or journalworthy acid reflux!

Having read the chapter on sleep and school performance already, you know the cycle these children fall into. They go to school late and subsequently stay up late, and the cycle is not healthy. While that problem is bad in and of itself, the addition of phones, laptops, televisions, and similar electronics adds a new dimension of danger for a variety of reasons.

Light

For most people, when it comes to modern electronics and sleep, their first concern is light. It is a valid concern. Light interferes with sleep. In fact, if you asked most sleep specialists, they would probably tell you that light is one of the biggest influencers on our sleep (and circadian timing in general).

So, ideally, a student goes to school every day in a bright, well-lit environment with as much exposure to the sun as possible (classrooms with big windows, eating lunch outside, getting some exercise outdoors, etc.). In the evening, as the sun goes down outside, that gradual loss of light is mirrored in the student's own living and sleep environment with limited TV and electronics in the thirty minutes to an hour before bed.

That's the ideal. Now, let's look at the real world. If a student makes it to school on time, the light they are exposed to in the morning and the light in the school is variable and often inadequate for optimal wakefulness. For kids who go to school virtually, there are some who awaken, log into class, mute their microphone, and turn off their video camera, and go back to sleep.* On the weekends, many kids sleep in, significantly.† Even when they are awake, many children linger in dark rooms. No outdoor exposure, no exercise, no light in general.

Suddenly the main source of light in a child's life is not the G-type main-sequence star of superheated plasma we call the sun, but rather a phone screen. These screens are actively harming our kids' ability to sleep and rest effectively. Why? Because they are tricking their brains into thinking that the sun is always up, and the process via which this works is fascinating.

First, understand that our brains are really in tune to both light amounts (bright day, cloudy day) as well as light change (slowly getting darker or brighter). If we all lived a camping existence (exclusively living outdoors and always being in an environment of slowly changing light with no other light contamination), I suspect many people would see shocking improvements to their sleep. Being a part of an environment that features lighting levels with consistent timing is very helpful to the

---

* We've come so far from the days of just putting your head down on the desk and nodding off anytime we hear the words "electoral college."

† The radically different weekday and weekend schedules lead to what has been dubbed "social jet lag."

brain in terms of knowing what time it is.* As someone who knows about circadian rhythms now, you are aware of how light forms the backbone of your child's circadian rhythm. But you may not be aware of the mechanics involved with making that happen.

When we are exposed to light that is both sufficient in intensity and quality, the light is detected by specialized cells in our eyes (in our retinas specifically). These cells in turn let our brains know about the light situation. The information is passed to our suprachiasmatic nucleus (SCN), the control center of our circadian rhythm. The SCN sends a signal to our pineal body/gland,† which in turn produces melatonin.

You will recall melatonin from chapter 3. Melatonin is a hormone that regulates the sleep wake cycle as it relates to our circadian rhythm. It is our brain's equivalent of the car's timing belt. It is not so much related to facilitating sleep as it is regulating the timing of one's sleep in relation to light/dark cycles outside. When we suppress melatonin with light, we feel less driven to sleep. When we facilitate the release of melatonin by being in the dark, we feel more driven to sleep.

That's all great for the prehistoric cave dweller or contestant on History Channel's riveting survival show *Alone*, but what if you are someone who does not live on a sporadic diet of available berries and smoked rabbit? There is lighting everywhere, and the screen in front of your child's face at night is producing a lot of it. So much so that it is fooling his brain into thinking it is lunchtime when it is really bedtime.

When we think about harmful light, we want to think about the amount of light being produced, and the wavelengths of light being emitted (the quality). You are probably already familiar with this to some degree. When you choose a light bulb, you may pay attention to the lumens listed on the packaging as an indicator of brightness. Back in the day, we just looked at the wattage of the typical incandescent bulb we were purchasing and knew 100-watt bulbs were really bright, and 60-watt

---

* Remember zeitgebers?

† Or epiphysis cerebri, if you still wear a toga.

bulbs were less so. Today we use lumens to measure the light output potential of a bulb.* For example, with the old incandescent bulbs:

40-watt bulb = 450 lumens
60-watt bulb = 800 lumens
75-watt bulb = 1,100 lumens
100-watt bulb = 1,600 lumens
150-watt bulb = 2,600 lumens

There is another measurement of which you should be aware. Besides the output of a bulb, there is actual light available in a specific area or environment. Specifically,

$$1 \text{ lux} = 1 \text{ lumen per 1 square meter}$$

In other words, imagine being in a totally dark museum and trying to look at Van Gogh's *Starry Night* painting hanging on the wall. That painting is roughly one square meter in size. Your friend has luckily brought a flashlight with her.† Imagine you are standing next to the painting, and your friend is shining that light on the wall from far across the room. The painting would be illuminated, but just barely. You can make out the general forms, but the details are obscured by the dim illumination. Now imagine your friend walking closer to you, all the while still shining the light on the painting you are studying. What happens with the light on the masterpiece? The light starts to become brighter and more concentrated. The colors come alive and the details reveal themselves as the light becomes brighter because the flashlight is closer. While

---

* I always notice these numbers when I look at the flashlights on display at the Home Depot checkout. I have absolutely no need for a 100,000 lumens flashlight in my life, but maybe I do. How would I know for sure without purchasing it and having it? Tragically, my wife always vetoes that purchase.

† Her partner allows her to buy any flashlight she wants, which is really cool.

the lumens rating of the flashlight never changes, the light intensity, or lux, at the painting got much higher as the light source got closer.

We can measure light intensity fairly easily. If you have ever watched a professional photographer at work, she will often use a handheld lux meter to measure the amount of light at the site of what she is photographing. You can pick up a lux meter for less than $100, and there are even some cell phone apps that do the job by using the phone's camera.

I know you are wondering why on earth we are talking about photography equipment when we came here to talk about your kid's sleep and nocturnal computer usage! It all boils down to how much light is passing through our pupils at various times of the day and night, and understanding how it affects our wakefulness and ability to achieve quality sleep. Magazine articles on sleep talk about this all the time, but they never get down to the nuts and bolts of how to know what is going on specifically in your home, and what to do about it. Well, here we go.

There are many studies looking at the light intensity needed to affect sleep. In general, studies utilize light sources of different magnitudes to help individuals maintain wakefulness, like in the example of a shift worker. In the middle of the night, that worker might intentionally expose themselves to a bright light in an effort to suppress melatonin secretion and wake up. Studies have shown that LED light sources of 2,000 lux or more to be highly effective in promoting wakefulness.

Conversely, there have been some studies attempting to identify the smallest amounts of light necessary to disrupt sleep. In one study, light amounts as low as 5 to 10 lux were enough to measurably disrupt the sleep of the young men and women in the study.* Regardless of the size of the screen, its mere presence in your child's room reduces their nightly sleep time by an average of eighteen to twenty minutes every night. This is the equivalent of losing fifteen nights of sleep every year. In the study, participants exposed to the light equivalent of a cell phone had significantly less sleep and more wakefulness during the night. While these studies have not been conducted in children, there is no reason to think that they would be immune to the effects of the light from electronics at night.

---

* This would be roughly the light level of a phone on night mode.

Up until this point, we have spoken solely of light intensity or brightness. Lux and lumens and cool flashlights are great, but there is another aspect of light that should be considered when we think about its impact of sleep: the quality of the light, or more specifically, what wavelengths make up the visible light we see.

If you remember back to science class in school, you may recall studying the properties of visible light. If you were not that into school, it is okay. Maybe Pink Floyd is more your thing. If so, picture *The Dark Side of the Moon* album cover and the prism refracting the white light into the color spectrum. What that prism is actually doing is separating out all the wavelengths of light that make up that beam of white light.

Today, more than ever, the wavelengths of light that make up the output from a bulb are very important. These light "ingredients" can be manipulated to produce different variations or temperatures of lighting. This lighting property is often referred to as color temperature. You are probably aware of this when you pick out light bulbs. "Warm," "cool," "natural," "soft," or "daylight" may be descriptors you have seen used for lighting. What do they mean, and how does it relate to sleep? It is really absorbing. At the risk of going too far afield, let's just look at the basics of color temperature.

The light bulb was invented when Thomas Edison figured out how to heat a filament enough to produce visible light. Pretty much everything we know emits heat. You and I do . . . a little anyway, and you can see it with an infrared camera (infrared energy is energy that is less than the energy of the color red—hence infrared). If we could control our body heat like a Marvel superhero and heat ourselves up to higher and higher levels, we would start to glow red. Why red? Because it is the lowest-energy color on the visible light spectrum . . . our heat would go from invisible infrared energy to visible red energy.

But superhero ability to raise our temperature does not stop there. When necessary, we can raise our temperature even further and heat our body up to unbelievable levels, so as the heat increases, our red color would start to become more orange . . . then white. But we are not done, still more heat . . . and now we begin to glow the familiar color blue. We are glowing blue because the increasing heat is now creating so much energy that we are moving into the higher energy level of the visible light spectrum.

Back to Thomas Edison. He's invented the light bulb. Now came the question: How hot should the filament be heated to get the most light for the least energy? At lower levels of energy/heat (2,000 kelvin), the light had a softer, warmer light that glowed more yellow. At higher temperatures (4,000 kelvin), the light looked whiter or natural. At even higher temperatures (5000+), the light looked more like daylight on a hot day . . . even taking on a blue hue.

These hues can be measured. The different amounts of "color" that make up any given light source can be measured and graphed by spectral power distribution. Think of this as how much blue or yellow or green color is being emitted by any given light.

In a typical incandescent bulb, while a full color spectrum is being produced the incandescent bulb's energy is heating it to the point where it is giving off far more red light than say blue (a softer light). When compared to the spectral analysis of pure daylight, it is clear that this bulb is not delivering nearly the same amount of blue light as natural morning or afternoon light.

Turning our attention to fluorescent and energy-efficient bulbs we see a very different pattern of color emission. The relative linear distribution of light is gone, and for these energy-efficient bulbs, discreet bands of some colors are produced with near absence of other colors. For example, the energy-efficient bulb has massive amounts of orange and lime green, but little else. Despite the strange mixture of colors, when the bulb gets turned on in your child's school or bedroom, all anyone sees is (1) white light, and (2) lower electricity bills.

While cinematographers, interior designers, and lighting specialists think about lighting temperature, color, and intensity a tremendous amount, the average parent of a child probably does not.* Previously, the decision basically boiled down to 100-watt bulbs where you needed lots

* Compare the Tatooine scenes from *Star Wars: A New Hope* to the Hoth scenes from *The Empire Strikes Back* for a great contrasting use of warm lighting to create a sense of heat to cool to create a sense of cold. For younger readers who are more

of light, and maybe a 60-watt bulb when you were trying to create a more relaxed and soothing atmosphere. No color choices (except for those weird yellow bulbs they used to sell), and no energy-efficient options. If you wanted to save energy, you went around the house turning lights off and griping about wasting money like my father when we were growing up. Much has changed.

Today, the options are endless but very important, because the light we choose to expose our children to can dramatically impact their sleep. In the world of sleep and wakefulness, this primarily has to do with the color *blue*, because it is this particular wavelength of light that affects the production of melatonin in your child's brain. When your child is exposed to a source of blue light (or a source of what appears to be white light with a high proportion of blue in its spectral analysis), the blue light strongly stimulates those retina receptors. These receptors measure signal intensity and trigger the suprachiasmatic nucleus, which in turn creates melatonin release from the pineal body. The more blue light, the more dramatic this effect.

For healthy sleep, ideally your child is literally bathing in ample blue light once she awakens and experiences a slow loss of blue light leading up to bedtime. This loss can occur as an overall loss of full spectrum (all of the visible colors) in the form of diminishing lux of light with a sunrise, or it can occur as a specific loss of blue light as your child approaches bedtime.

For the cave dweller, or family living totally off the grid, this is no problem. As you are eating your dinner outside, the sun slowly begins to drop in the sky. As the night fills the space, you might read a few pages by the dwindling campfire before you decide to call it a night. Most sleep researchers believe that this is the way our bodies were intended to sleep.

This is a difficult environment to achieve in the modern household, and in many ways this has little to do with technology. Modern lighting is everywhere and prevents our brains from typically "seeing" the

---

familiar with *Game of Thrones*, you can substitute Yunkai for Tatooine and Castle Black for Hoth.

sunset. Our society runs twenty-four hours a day, so there are not as many cues to let us know the day is ending. However, you have the power to change this.

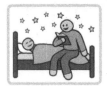 Wow, you made it through some pretty technical stuff. I hope you found it somewhat interesting and enjoyable. If you did, great. If you didn't, well, it is over and time to use the information you have gathered to make some impactful changes.

I'm going to suggest you make a couple purchases. First, I want you to purchase a digital light meter. Nothing fancy. I just saw one on Amazon for about $20. We discussed this device earlier as the item photographers use to determine the amount of light (measured in lux) at a given spot in space. With this device, you will be able to determine exactly how much light is reaching a certain point (like your daughter's desk where she does homework in the evening, or her bed where she sleeps at night). I really don't like asking people to fork out money, but I think you will really enjoy using this. I also think that if you have kids, this would be a great device to use as a basis for a science fair project. Perhaps you could rent the device to others for a small fee so that they can do lighting assessments of their homes, schools, and places of work.

Second, grab one more item: a spectroscope (sometimes called a spectrometer). These usually run about $10–$40 depending on the design. The one I own looks like a tiny telescope. Remember the spectral analyses of light we discussed earlier? Well, this device can help you determine the relative amounts of different wavelengths of light coming from the various sources of light in your home, and it is as easy to use as looking through a microscope!

Okay, now you are fully equipped to do a full lighting assessment of your home, school, or place of work!

First, I want you to play around with your light meter and get to know how it works. Walk around your house and take some measurements to get a feel for various light levels. For example, I've taken some daytime readings from a dark corner of my basement (259 lux), my living room near a window (4,010 lux), and outside on a deck (16,470 lux).

Notice the dramatically different measurements you are getting in different areas . . . 100 lux, 1,000 lux, 10,000 lux; all depending on where you are standing in the home. Now take your device and stand away from a light source like a lamp or a window. Look how dramatically your readings can change based upon your proximity to the light source. This is a great example of the difference between lumens and lux. The light source (lumens) of the lamp is not changing; however, the light exposure (lux) you are measuring with your light meter increases steadily as you get closer to the source.

Now that you are familiar with the device and the relative light levels of the house, here is the important part: what light level should your kids be exposed to to feel their best during the day and sleep their best at night? Before we begin, let's set some guideposts. For the sake of this conversation, let's call sitting outside in a chair doing work on a sunny day 10,000 lux (my reading of 16,470 lux was in fact taken on a deck at the Phillies spring training facility in Clearwater, Florida, on a very bright day). And let's call total darkness 0 lux.

For kids, research tells us that an environment with a lux level of 5,000 lux or more is most ideal for promoting wakefulness. Generally, the minimum recommended light to effectively see in a classroom is 300 lux, but generally 500–1,000 optimal for routine classwork, and 1,500–2,000 lux for detailed work. On the flip side, we know that as little as 5 lux can disrupt sleep. With your light meter, you can now see what conditions your kids are in when they are eating dinner, doing homework, and sleeping at night. More important, if they are not serving your child's needs, you can fix it!

Ideally, there should be a steady loss of light in your child's environment from dinner to bedtime. After dinner, walk outside with your light meter and take a reading. What does it say? I just went outside and did this. It is 6:42 p.m., and outside on my deck, I got a reading of 1,061 lux. Next, I check on my kids. My daughter, a college student, is doing work in her bedroom. The light reading was 37 lux. My son was in front of a laptop in a brightly lit basement. That reading was 2,210 lux.

It is important to establish the desired goal of an individual working in a given lighting environment. If both my kids want to work productively for a few hours and then go to sleep, are they setting themselves up for that to happen?

As the evening progresses and the light outdoors gradually diminishes, if both children maintain the same circumstances, I suspect that my daughter will soon grow weary of her reading and want to go to sleep. As she feels tired, if sleep is not an option, perhaps she will seek caffeine, or some snacks to help wake up. A big question in this situation is whether the quality of her work will shift as concentration and focus begin to drift.

Conversely, my son is going to feel far more energized in his situation given the substantial lighting to which he is exposed. For him, as the time he wants to retire draws closer, if he does not begin to diminish the light level intensity in his environment, he runs the risk of having difficulty falling asleep when the time comes.

Here is where you come in. With a light meter, you can help control the lighting to which your children are exposed. Have interested kids? Talk to them about what you are doing. Are your kids young or not interested, or you just enjoy experimenting on them? That's okay too. Walk into your daughter's room and turn on another light. Head down to the basement and turn off the bright overhead lights for a dimmer desk light. Need a home improvement project? Buy some dimmer switches this weekend and install them everywhere your kids are in the evening and control the light. After dinner, create a sunset inside your home that slowly reduces that light level to 0 when your child is in bed.

Light quantity level reduction: check. But that's only half the battle against light at night.* There is still quality to think about, and because of that second purchase, you can actually see what wavelengths your child is being exposed to . . . and remediate it. There are several ways to remove blue light, or more broadly blue-green light specifically in the 450–525 nanometer wavelength range, the wavelength thought to suppress sleep the most.

---

* Maybe more than half the battle, as a recent study in *Current Biology* by Tim Brown and others suggests that the intensity of the light plays a far bigger role at night than the light quality.

THREE WAYS TO GET RID OF SLEEP-HARMING WAVELENGTHS OF
LIGHT

1. You can eliminate all visible light, which gets rid of everything
from 380–700 nanometers.

2. You can eliminate specific wavelengths of light.

3. You can filter out specific wavelengths of light.

All these represent viable options. Option #1 is the light/dimmer
switch, or simply turning off or reducing sources of light in your child's
immediate environment prior to sleeping. It's cheap, pretty easy, and anyone can turn off or dim a light.

Option #2 involves purchasing lighting that does not have the sleep-
inhibiting blue light we are concerned about. These bulbs are great options
for a kid's bedroom where he may be up studying at night. Once you've
decided what bulb to purchase, take a look at it with your new spectroscope. Is it really emitting less blue-green light than a standard bulb?

Another way to eliminate specific wavelengths of light is via our home
electronics. Many laptops and phones have "sleep modes" that do this for
us. By selecting this mode, the blue-green light emitted by the screen
disappears and the display takes on a pinkish hue. There are free apps
like f.lux that can be downloaded to accomplish this task if your laptop
does not have these settings.

Option #3 is to leave the light in your home or bedrooms as it is, and
instead utilize a filter to prevent it from reaching your retinas. The easiest filter to purchase is blue-blocking glasses. For about $10, you can buy
some glasses that look like something Bono wears in concert, and stick
them on your child's face as he sails a virtual pirate ship or whatever he's
doing in his gaming world. These glasses are typically yellow, and your
child might complain about his world suddenly looking more lemony,
but he'll adjust. More important, the game he's playing at night or the
evening YouTube videos will not have as negative of an impact on his
sleep without the blue light reaching his face.

Stress, Addiction, and Dopamine

The light emitted by electronics is harmful. There is no doubt that lighting in general plays a significant role in the sleep of all ages of kids. But lighting has been around for a while. I'm sure some village group back in time was protesting about the hidden dangers of nocturnal torchlight. With electronics, the sleep problems go much deeper than a new source of environmental light and strike at the very seat of motivation and addiction in the brains of our children.

If you think about the primitive neural circuitry of an earthworm, it seems vastly different from the brain of the child living in your home. One thing that these two living things share is goal-directed activity.* You can make an argument that everything we do is goal directed, particularly if you happen to be an earthworm. There are several ways to group goals: short-term (eat food), intermediate (prepare for a big dinner party this weekend), and long-term (I need to consume a healthier diet). You can also group them in terms of their reward payout: immediate big reward (eat a pizza that was just delivered) versus delayed—have a piece of sourdough bread that you baked using a starter you have been cultivating and feeding for weeks.

At the center of this reward is the chemical dopamine. This is an important neurotransmitter in our brains, and it is involved in many things our brains control: movement, mood, and motivation. When our brains do something that is pleasurable, the reward pathway runs through dopamine, and it makes us feel good.

Outside of movement, mood, and motivation, there is another big function of dopamine, and unfortunately it does not begin with *M*, because that would be way too easy and cool. It is sleep! Well, actually it's wakefulness, but they are related. Here's how:

Remember those curves from chapter 1? I'll repeat one here to illustrate how dopamine works in the body. Like just about everything else, dopamine has a circadian rhythm. As you've learned, a circadian rhythm has a predictable daily biological pattern of function or behavior. In this

* #goals if you are a kid.

graph, the line represents dopamine levels in the body over the period of a day. Notice how they tend to peak around lunchtime and then begin to fall until around midnight, when they reach rock bottom and begin to rise again.

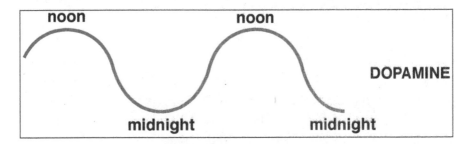

By looking at this graph, I'll bet you can guess how dopamine affects wakefulness and sleepiness. Dopamine helps us feel awake and engaged, which is why it is generally high during the day* and tends to drop off at night. Playing around with curves, what do you think would be the sleep consequence in an individual who did not make much dopamine?

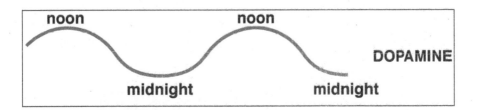

Correct. They would be sleepy all the time. And this is what is seen in adults (and kids) who have Parkinson's disease or symptoms of parkinsonism. The cells that produce dopamine stop working properly and

---

* One might assume by looking at this graph that our wakefulness would peak around lunchtime. This may seem at odds with the feeling we might get around lunchtime that we want to take a nap. The truth is that dopamine is not the only neurotransmitter involved with wakefulness, and it is the other neurotransmitters and chemicals that rescue us from the tremendous crash that would occur if dopamine were solely responsible for wakefulness. Because of this system, while we don't crash, some of us do feel the dip!

dopamine levels fall, creating many problems including significant sleep issues. Keep in mind, these same problems can be seen in kids who take dopamine-blocking medications like Thorazine (chlorpromazine), Reglan (metoclopramide), Phenergan (promethazine), Risperdal (risperidone), Seroquel (quetiapine), and Clozaril (clozapine), commonly used in some psychiatric or neurological disorders.

I know what you are thinking. I thought this chapter was about *Call of Duty* and TikTok videos. It is . . . we are almost there! Now, let's continue to theorize about dopamine and its relationship to sleep. If a drop in dopamine is sleep promoting and a rise is sleep inhibiting, it would make sense that we want to facilitate that natural fall in dopamine that escorts us all into a perfect night of sleep. Agreed? Great.

Now knowing what you know about dopamine, which of the following seems most pro-dopamine for a fourteen-year-old boy in the hour leading up to bedtime?

- An attractive TikTok influencer or his girlfriend preening in a bikini on their iPhone.

- A violent video game where he is trying to infiltrate an abandoned compound and take out the paramilitary troops occupying the installation.

- A thrilling semifinal basketball game played at home in front of his classmates/school that goes into double overtime with his team seizing the victory on a buzzer-beating three-pointer.

- Quietly reading a non-school book in bed illuminated only by the soft lighting of a reading lamp.

Ignoring exercise like playing a basketball game—which is awesome but also very dopamine-productive (and it's why many athletes have trouble "coming down" after a big game)—let's focus on the TikTok influencer and her dance video as well as the violent video game. Look, I'm not here to bash either of these forms of entertainment. I have played video games before* and have consumed and produced social media. It is not so much the *what*, but rather the *when*. Swiftly sweeping an abandoned warehouse looking for zombies or enemy combatants who are trying to murder you all the while shooting others and taking their belongings is great fun, but imagine the surge of dopamine these kinds of images and activities are producing.

> Bam! Bam! Bam! The sniper is dead and you get to steal his gun and ammo.
>
> —immediate release of dopamine—
>
> Attractive individual who conveniently forgot to fully dress does a quick provocative dance to "Tap In."
>
> —immediate release of dopamine—
>
> While playing *Grand Theft Auto*, you rob a bank, take hostages, and end the day by soliciting a prostitute that you may or may not murder to get your money back.†
>
> —double dose.

Okay, now it is 10:00 p.m. and bedtime. Charge your phone downstairs and go to bed, dear.

Good luck with that!

After one exciting, exhilarating, titillating video or game after another, not to mention the light being emitted from the screen, your child's dopamine is soaring. They are wide awake now and currently frustrated that the funny videos of kids eating spoonfuls of cinnamon have come to an end for the evening. Their brains are racing as they look for the next "hit" of excitement.

---

* I prefer pinball . . . old-school.

† This is a real game that little kids are exposed to. I know this because the twelve-year-old brother of a patient was playing it in the exam room while I took care of his sibling.

I'm not causally using the word "hit" here. Make no mistake that these devices and games act like a drug to your kids. Whether it is a hit of cocaine or a hit of *Call of Duty*, the only difference is the relative amount of dopamine produced. Now the problem becomes apparent:

If dopamine produces wakefulness and facilitates addiction . . .

And if TV, video games, cell phones, etc., produce a dramatic dopaminergic response . . .

Then:

1. Kids are becoming addicted to their phones and computers, which is no surprise because they are designed to facilitate and encourage addiction.

2. The use of these devices and media will promote wakefulness if utilized at night, which happens to be the time kids have free to play since it is tough to play *Mario Kart* during AP US History.

So right when we want to facilitate the drop in dopamine that we see naturally occurring after lunch, that iPhone in your daughter's back pocket is delivering a huge amount of alerting dopamine to her brain.

This sets up a conflict. A parent armed with concern, and love, and science along with a child who wants to do better in math, feel less anxious, and do the right thing is *no match* for an app designed by an intelligent programmer to push your son's dopamine button repeatedly when he plays.

My point with electronics and sleep is both simple and impossible. The simple part is that yes, these devices are hurting your kid's sleep. A 2016 retrospective literature review of screen time in school-aged children found an overwhelmingly significant association (90 percent) between screen time and diminished sleep, to the point that the authors seem to state that scientists can stop trying to prove if the relationship exists and instead focus on trying to determine how big of a problem we have on our hands.

Simple solution, right? We, as parents, will just take their phones and laptops away or significantly limit our kid's exposure. I have probably bellowed something to this effect on a weekly basis since 2010. While this is a perfectly easy idea to say (or write), it is significantly harder to put this plan into action as numerous obstacles are in the way.

The technology is ubiquitous. I mean, it is literally everywhere, and if your children attend public schools, you can almost forget about it. Today, many schools issue or require students to have tablets. As a parent, you may simply not allow your children to have it, I suppose, but every aspect of the student's life is funneled through that device. Assignments are on the computer. Communications are via the computer. Grades are posted on the computer.* Classes occur virtually via the computer. If the COVID-19 crisis has taught us anything, it is that the computer is now more important than the actual brick-and-mortar school your kids attend. Today, the computer essentially is your child's school.

Your kids know more about the technology than you and the guy at the Verizon office. To me, this is a huge problem. I have no issues with phones. They help keep my kids safe and in communication with me when we are separated. Being able to look at my phone and see where my kids are is very helpful and reassuring. It would be great if we could limit the time kids spend on their phones and the types of activities in which they involve themselves while on the phones, but I increasingly think that is impossible. I'm pretty sure that if you were to approach a group of middle schoolers and say "parental controls," they would all spontaneously start to laugh. My kids (who are by no means elite computer hacker–types) easily find their way around parental controls, passwords that we install on devices, blocked apps, and other safeguards. I'm certain that the same is true for that "safe" tablet they receive from school.

The benefits of technology. In a similar way that the sugar industry

---

* And grades are emailed/texted to parents. Wow, what a blessing and a curse when at 2:00 p.m. I received a text notifying me that my child has a D in his math class. This leads to some kind of communication or confrontation in which my child says that the D is not real because he did not turn in two assignments because he missed class because of a jazz band field trip and he's already emailed the teacher about it. Sometimes one can have too much information.

was able to wield its financial muscle to block, misdirect, and obscure the dangers of sugar and keep the public in the dark about the dangers of consuming too much of it, I assume the technology industry is doing the same. When it comes to sleep, technology, and children, I have read items here and there suggesting, for example, that video games are good for children. It is improving their attention. See how Tommy really struggles with attention in school but can sit in front of his television all weekend playing *Star Wars Battlefront* on his Xbox?

In reality, these devices tend to negatively affect children and their attention over time. Video games have been described as misguided or failed attempts by kids to self-medicate their attention issues with the dopamine surges associated with scoring virtual touchdowns or killing virtual enemy combatants—this provocative and lurid content being a necessary ingredient for the process to work. The child needs more video games over time to ease his anxiety. He needs more graphic content, more action, more bells and whistles . . . why?

Because social media and video games are essentially drugs when it comes to your child's brain. And what do drug users need over time? More drugs and more intense highs. Here are just some of the behaviors I have seen from kids looking for their next video game fix:

- bargaining;

- tantrums;

- using devices like school calculators to download and play games;

- secretly getting game devices from friends;

- reactivating old cell phones around the house that have been replaced;

- creating fake phones out of wood to "plug in at night" while the real phone is in the bedroom with the child.

That last behavior is inspired by my youngest son, who would slip his phone out of his iPhone case, then flip the case facedown and plug it in.

When we looked over at our charging area, we saw his phone there, all plugged in and not in his room keeping him up at night. It took us months before my wife finally figured out that it was just an empty case.

If these behaviors seem like drug-seeking behaviors to you, it is because that is precisely what they are. Face it. If our kids could smash up an iPhone 10 into a fine powder and snort it, they would. This is what you are up against.

Fixing the Problem

One of my pet peeves with doctors is what I refer to as "the overreach." Here is an example:

> **Pediatrician:** "Your child is overweight. According to this graph
> in front of me, a child of his height should weigh 105 pounds.
> Your child weighs 145 pounds. He needs to lose forty pounds."
> **Parent:** "Uh sure. Okay."
> **Pediatrician:** "Wonderful, it was great seeing you both today."

The overreach involves seeing a patient in front of you and seeing a goal on the horizon, and instead of creating steps to reach that goal, one immediately jumps to the goal with no well-formulated plan to get there. As frustration happens, failure soon sets in.

I'm a sleep specialist, not a technology mitigator. Having said that, there are some concrete steps you can take to get control of your child's technology use and prevent it from affecting her sleep.

Don't let it start. If I'm too late with this advice, ignore it. But if you are reading this book with a baby in your partner's belly, it's never too early to formalize your electronics plan. Remember when we talked about getting an early start in terms of things a mother can do to be laying the groundwork for good sleep even before the delivery? Those same ideas can apply to technology.

How will you use technology in your life? Will your child be exposed to television programs, and starting at what age? When during the day will these programs be consumed? Will a phone or television privileges be given to a child only during specific times, or anytime things are boring like in waiting rooms and trips to the post office? When will parents be on their own phones?

Starting now, develop clearly defined rules for technology in your child's life. Here are several definitive steps you can take to start to gain control of the situation.

- **Out in the open.** Consider having children play games or interact on the computer/phone in an environment where they can be seen, utilizing headphones. Parents are often quite shocked by the subject matter of the games their children are playing. Having it out in the open can be a much healthier situation.

- **Limit game-playing time.** We want our children to lead lives that are healthy and diverse. Electronics often give kid's brains a sense of accomplishment when there in fact is none . . . just the manipulation of light patterns on a screen. Games and TikTok scrolling are like those junky breakfast cereals . . . not part of a well-balanced diet. Electronics should be a small part of a well-balanced life in children that might include things like academics, athletics, real social interaction with friends and family, spirituality, volunteerism, playing an instrument, personal care, and sleep. Maybe your child does not need all these items in their life, but all too often the phone becomes a disproportionately large part of the pie.

- **Pre-bedtime moratorium.** Ideally for children, they should be off devices two hours before bedtime. If school does not allow this to happen, take steps to limit the light your child is exposed to by utilizing blue-blocking glasses.

- **Phones sleep in the kitchen, stay out of the bedroom.** Make it a rule for everyone that phones and laptops sleep in the kitchen. This goes for parents too. Create a space with chargers and outlets that clearly allows anyone to see whose phone is present (just watch out for the case-only trick!), and whose is absent.

When phones are in use, limit their use in the bedroom. Keep that space reserved for sleep and sleep-promoting activities as much as possible.

- **Don't let phones be your children's alarms.** I'm not sure if your kids are aware of this, but we had alarm clocks prior to cell phones. They wound up and had little bells on top. Anna Steese Richardson can tell you all about them. Purchase a stand-alone alarm for your kids. I'm particularly fond of the alarms that utilize light to awaken kids in the morning. For more stubborn sleepers, consider alarms that shake the bed or require purposeful interactions before they can be shut off.

- **Go to the source.** Utilize the parental limits on your kids' phones and wireless internet. Your kids are smart, but the woman at Verizon is smarter (hopefully!). Let her show you how to cut your kids off by shutting off the wireless internet or using password-protected media limits on your child's phone. Make it a rule to frequently check their usage amounts, and discuss it with them. My kids are usually pretty shocked when we look at how many minutes they spent on their devices.

 I would like to say that Tiffany's story had a happy, breezy ending. It did not. It was complicated, messy, and involved a lot of work. Despite my relatively small and discreet role as "the sleep doctor," the family continued to follow up with me on a regular basis. Dr. Ivan Login, a neurologist at the University of Virginia and one of the many neurologists who trained me, once said, "Sometimes having the answer is less important than just listening to the problem."

Things started slowly. Step one was simply eliminating the gaming at night. While that seems quite simple and logical on the surface, the removal of the video games seemed to either cause or unearth very significant issues related to social anxiety, self-worth, and feelings of control.

"I control my world in *Minecraft*, and I control who I am inside of it. I like that world better." For Tiffany, the choice was an idealized world with an idealized Tiffany inside it, or going to bed and waking up to a reality that was, in her mind, bordering on traumatic.

With time, Tiffany improved. She never ended up having a sleep study, although we considered it several times and always kept the option open. Tiffany currently lives on her own, works, and attends a local community college where she studies computer science and wants to design video games that improve health and sleep rather than take away from it.

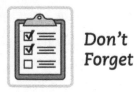 **Don't Forget**

1. Modern electronics pose a significant threat to the sleep of our children.

2. Video games and social media, due to the addictive content they provide, can be especially harmful to children getting the requisite amount of sleep.

3. With the right equipment, you can make positive changes in the lighting character and intensity your kids are exposed to, and subsequently improve sleep and wakefulness naturally.

4. It is up to you to understand the content of the media your child consumes and put appropriate limits on it. There is no such thing as starting this process too early.

Nightmares, Night Terrors, Sleepwalking and -talking and -eating

More Nighttime Drama and Screaming than a Real Housewives *Episode*

 Jamie was a first-year college student at the University of Virginia. She and her parents made the nearly nine-hour trek from her home in Toledo, Ohio, all the way to Charlottesville, Virginia, to get her moved into her dorm. After the last trunk was wheeled in, the bed was made, and roommates were introduced, Jamie's parents tearfully departed and began the long drive back to Ohio.

About a week after Jamie began school, her parents got a call around 3:00 a.m.

"Hi, Dad, it's Jamie. Can you come pick me up?" Jamie's voice was calm, clear, and very matter-of-fact.

"Jamie, it is three a.m. and we are in Toledo. What's wrong? Why do you need us to pick you up?" her father asked, a rising tone of panic in his voice.

"I'm just turned around and can't figure out where to go, but I'll just sort it out. Bye." She hung up the phone. Jamie's father immediately redialed the number, but there was no response, and it was not Jamie's number.

About an hour later, campus police found a slightly confused young woman trying to make a phone call with a police emergency phone. She was barefoot and dressed only in small shorts and a tank top. She seemed unclear about her name and was not sure where she lived. She was carrying no form of identification. Through patient questioning and deduction, they were able to figure out her dorm and get her back to her room. Remarkably, no intoxication charges were levied, nor was any medical workup requested at the time.

The day after the incident, Jamie had no recollection of any of the events when questioned by her resident adviser (RA). Her father was contacted by the RA, and an appointment was made for her in my office, although they were not exactly sure what they were asking me to evaluate.* They simply wrote the word "confused" on the consultation form.

Jamie was anything but confused. She was bright, participative, and seemed generally eager to get to the bottom of whatever this incident was that people were talking about but that she could not remember. Sensing the lead to be cold, I asked Jamie's permission to call her parents. She agreed, and I called. Her father answered, and when I introduced myself, he asked if Jamie had been sleepwalking again.

"Again?" I asked. "Has she done this before?"

"Absolutely. At least once a week since she could walk."

~ ~ ~

Sleep is supposed to be a time of peaceful, quiet recovery, though for many, it is anything but. For centuries, literature and art have romanticized the terrors of the night, giving us glimpses of demonic possessions, visiting succubi, or any number of horrifying nightmares. For people who struggle with these disorders though, the phenomena are anything

---

* "Send them to the neurologist" is a common move when nobody has a clue about what is going on with a patient.

but romantic. And if you happen to be the parent of a child who has difficulty in this arena, you likely experience the night on eggshells, wondering if your child will act out in some concerning way.

Parasomnias

To understand what these disorders are, it is helpful to first define them. Parasomnias are a group of undesirable sleep disorders that involve seemingly purposeful actions or events that occur during various stages of sleep, particularly during sleep-wake transitions. Generally, they are characterized and defined by (1) the nature of the action (e.g., walking, talking, eating), (2) the timing of the action (e.g., during dream sleep, during deep sleep), and (3) a child's memory and insight into the event. Because memory of the disorder may not be present, parasomnias occurring in children are often not detected.

The bad news is that approximately 50 percent of children will experience some form of parasomnia, as these are among the most common sleep disorders in children. The good news is these disorders tend not to follow children into adulthood, as only 4 percent of parasomnias persist past adolescence.

Sleep Talking (Somniloquy)

Sleep talking is a good place to start, because it is the most common parasomnia—so common that some sleep researchers feel it can be a normal part of sleeping if it only happens occasionally.* Generally, sleep talking happens in the first half of the night, during the time that deep sleep is most prevalent. Sometimes it happens so quickly that it seems like your child may simply be singing in his room, arguing with a sibling, or innocently talking to herself. When somniloquy happens during deep sleep, the language is often garbled and unintelligible. This is in contrast to sleep talking that occurs during REM sleep, which is more common in the second half of the night. Language spoken during REM

---

* Think of it like sneezing. Every now and then, it's no big deal. But sneezing hundreds of times each day would be something to discuss with your allergist.

sleep is often more understandable and meaningful, and it's often re-membered the following day.

While talking in your sleep is seen in both genders, it is more commonly reported in boys. In general, parasomnias of all types generally diminish over time, with most becoming near absent to fully absent by age thirteen. Sleep talking is a bit of an exception to this general parasomnia rule of extinction. In some cases, it can persist into adulthood, or in rare cases, begin later in adolescence or adulthood. Often if this occurs or the sleep talking is escalating in frequency or intensity, this can be a sign that more aggressive intervention may be necessary.

More than any parasomnia, there is often the perception that your child's sleep talking is related to their mood or to particular events occurring in the home. It is understandable to think that one might draw a relationship between nocturnal screaming and emotional unrest. While there is an association between underlying anxiety and sleep talking, it has never been proven to be a causal relationship. In other words, while the two seem to travel together, there is no evidence that the anxiety is causing the sleep talking. Adversity has also not been linked to sleep talking, so the argument you had with your son over video games or your daughter's distress over a Latin exam does not make it more likely that sleep talking will occur.

The decision to address somniloquy is always up to the parent. If it does not seem to be affecting the health and well-being of your child, and it is not distressing you or siblings, it is perfectly fine not to address it and continue to monitor for any changes. If it is something that becomes disruptive or violent, socially awkward, or indicative that something else might be happening, a visit with a sleep specialist is never inappropriate.

Sleepwalking (Somnambulism)

With sleepwalking, we move from a parasomnia that is considered a normal variant to a parasomnia that falls squarely into the category of abnormal. These behaviors arise from sudden but incomplete arousals from deep sleep. A sleepwalker's actions and behaviors are typically inappropriate, and their recollection of the event is either partial or absent altogether. The lack of memory of a particular nocturnal event is a hallmark of somnambulism in children; as kids mature, there may start to be vague and incomplete recollections of "something happening" last night.

As many as 17 percent of children will sleepwalk, with the vast majority growing out of it prior to adulthood. Two to 4 percent of adults will sleepwalk. The vast majority of these adults were in fact sleepwalkers as kids. It is unusual and concerning when adults suddenly begin to ambulate at night with no confirmed history of sleepwalking as a child. As such, sleepwalking seems to be highly genetic and can often run in families. Kids of sleepwalkers are ten times more likely to be sleepwalkers themselves. When I see a child who is a sleepwalker, the first question I ask is about the biological parents and whether they were sleepwalkers as well.

These events typically occur during the first half or even first third of the night. As with somniloquy, the rapidity with which they occur after sleep onset may lead a parent to think that the child never went to sleep and is walking around delaying bedtime.

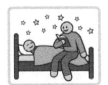

Treating somnambulism is difficult, but there are things that can be done besides doing nothing, as is commonly the remedy.

Before we begin, it is very important to highlight that a common cause of parasomnias like sleepwalking is sleeping pill use, particularly Ambien. In a book about children, this should be a rare cause, but kids get prescribed many things and even have access to meds they were not prescribed. We want to be aware of everything.

Before any treatment begins, it is paramount to take immediate steps to ensure your child's safety in the situation. While the treatment of sleepwalking is going to involve dealing with the sleepwalking itself and looking for and addressing the cause, finding the underlying cause or best treatment can take time. So safety comes first. Steps need to be taken to ensure your child's safety in the bedroom during the treatment process.

First take a look at your child's room. Ideally it should be located on the first floor or on a basement level to minimize fall risk should she climb out a window or stumble on stairs. It is important to close and properly secure all windows; never permanently "lock" a window or make it impossible to open as this could have dire consequences in a fire or other emergency situation. On that note, a child should never be locked into a room or physically restrained in any way, as this may prevent egress from a room in emergency situations or increase the risk of strangulation.

Your child should always sleep in pajamas or other nightclothes and never sleep naked. If there is reason to suspect your child may be getting too hot or too cold at night, appropriate steps should be taken to ensure their clothes are not exacerbating the problems, as this could be a trigger for sleepwalking. The use of a top bunk is also discouraged, even though I have had parents suggest the difficulty in getting out of the bunk was a positive in terms of curbing somnambulism. I did once have a student patient who leaped out of their bunk and acquired a subdural hematoma when he struck his head on the nightstand, so proceed with caution. If a kid wants out of a top bunk at night, they are getting out, one way or another (dangerous) way!

There is so much bad advice circulating around about how to handle a sleepwalking child if you come across them in the act. "Don't wake them up! They will freak out!" or "Don't look directly into a sleepwalker's eyes, you'll turn to stone." It is hard to keep track of them all. Here's the deal: if you come across a kid you think is sleepwalking, relax. Evoke a tone in your voice that is very matter-of-fact . . . bored even. Play along a little if necessary. Just work to ease their confusion, frustration, irritation, or fear while working to get them back to bed.

"It is okay . . . you are home and safe. Let's get you back to bed."

"But the meeh fur gruhs are at the beez porly . . ."

"Yes, I know, and that's fine. I checked with everyone and they are all perfectly happy with the situation. We can sort it out in the morning. You're fine, you just need to rest. It is all under control." The one exception to this pseudo Jedi mind trick is if your child is attempting to leave the home or do something that might be physically harmful to herself or others. In those cases, judicious physical restraint may be necessary. Throughout the process, the suggestion of "Let's get you back to bed" should be quietly repeated.

Once appropriate safety measures have been taken, it is time to hopefully find a cause. Fortunately, there are several considerations. It is very important that your clinician work to rule all of them out. Before you embark on the search for the cause or treatment, you need to create a log of your child's sleepwalking. The log does not need to be elaborate. Filling it full of details will only confuse the clinician and the extra work will, over time, dampen your enthusiasm to keep the journal.

My suggestion is that it looks something like this:

Sunday	Monday	Tuesday	Wednesday	Thursday	Friday	Saturday
			2		2	1
2						3 (tried to leave house)
2		1			2	
1						2
2	1					

In this diary, a blank for a day means that Mom and Dad were not aware of their child's sleepwalking. A "1" is maybe hearing some talking, a "2" is definite movement in the room, and "3" is something determined to be a bit more severe or concerning (numerous episodes, screaming, or, as this example shows, attempting to leave the bedroom or home).

The point of the journal is to make it simple and very easy to read. I can quickly see that this month, twelve out of thirty-one nights featured irregular behavior (39 percent of nights). The average "severity score" on nights where behaviors were noted is 1.75. The average score for all nights was 0.7 (assuming a blank equals 0). I can see the patient went five nights without an observed episode twice during this period. I also get a sense that the events seem to cluster around the weekend with ten out of twelve events happening between Friday and Sunday.* Journals like this are not only remarkably helpful in terms of understanding baseline frequencies, patterns, and severity of behaviors, they are also essential in terms of monitoring the success or failure of treatments. Going from six episodes per week to four episodes per week is a big improvement, but sometimes it doesn't "feel" like it. Having a more objective account of what your child is up to is always useful.

Causes of Sleepwalking

When looking for a cause for sleepwalking, pay attention to timing. Has your child always seemed to sleepwalk, or is it a new activity? Has your older child done it consistently since they were young, or did it go away for a while and reappear? Keep these characteristics in mind as you work your way through these potential causes.

- First, take a hard look at the genetics of the situation. Do/did your child's biological siblings struggle with sleepwalking? How about you and your partner? What about your child's grandparents? Understanding the genetics and the clinical course that other family members experienced with their sleepwalking can be exceptionally helpful.

- While the connection between significant psychological disease (e.g., major depression, anxiety, bipolar mood disorder) or a major psychological stressor and sleepwalking is not strong, situational stress has been linked to sleepwalking. Taking steps to reduce stress before bedtime, eliminate disturbing images from television or other media, and working to create a more peaceful bedtime environment can be helpful.

---

* This is based on a real patient's diary who was having more events on the weekends and near the weekends because of sleep deprivation and staying up later on the weekends. The later nights made it hard for him to fall asleep on Sunday night.

- Additionally, sleep deprivation is a common trigger. Often the addition of as little as fifteen to thirty minutes added to the sleep period (preferably a bedtime fifteen to thirty minutes earlier rather than sleeping in an additional fifteen to thirty minutes) can markedly reduce sleepwalking occurrences.

- There is some evidence that suggests increased body temperature via either fever or nocturnal activity prior to bed can induce somnambulism. Taking steps to create a cooler sleeping environment for your child can be helpful. Studies have shown that nocturnal administration of acetaminophen and the resultant drop in body temperature result in reduced sleepwalking. Acetaminophen has the potential of dropping core body temperature by .1 to .4°C in normal subjects, so this can be useful even if your child does not have a fever. Prolonged exposure to acetaminophen can have negative health consequences particularly related to the liver and kidney. Consult your primary care physician or sleep specialist before starting any medication.

- Some medications might precipitate sleepwalking. These medications include:

  - benzodiazepines (Valium, Ativan, Prosom, Klonopin);

  - sodium oxybate (Xyrem);

  - zolpidcm (Ambien);

  - selective serotonin reuptake inhibitors (Prozac, Paxil, Zoloft, etc.).

If your child takes any of these medications, or you feel the start of the sleepwalking episodes corresponds with the onset of your child taking any drugs or supplements, discuss this with your physician immediately.

- Epilepsy and seizure disorders can present as sleepwalking or stereotyped behaviors (behaviors that are repetitive and abnormal) during the night.* An evaluation by a neurologist and/or epileptologist as well as an accompanying EEG may be appropriate.

- Other sleep disorders are common causes of sleepwalking. Addressing the presence of snoring, gastroesophageal reflux, periodic limb movement, or teeth grinding (bruxism) can often eliminate sleepwalking. Evaluation of these disorders may require a sleep study.

- There have been cases of psychiatric dissociative disorders presenting like sleepwalking at night. I intentionally put this last on the list because it irritates me when physicians jump right to this diagnosis without meticulously evaluating other possible causes. That said, sleepwalking can be seen in the cases of trauma (often sexual abuse) and present as conversion disorders. In these disorders, the patient will be aware of the sleepwalking episodes but may not admit it. While I'm certainly not against seeing a mental health specialist or counselor, I believe it is important to not jump directly to this option or put a significant amount of assumption into this being the ultimate solution. As mentioned before, the research linking psychiatric disorders and sleepwalking is thin at best.

Treating Primary Sleepwalking

I was hoping that you would not make it to this section because either your kid's sleepwalking magically disappeared, or something I wrote turned out to be the cause, and once addressed, things improved. That didn't happen. That's okay. It just means there is more to be done.

I'm using the term "primary" to denote this sleepwalking because I

---

* The classic sleep conference example is a patient who awakens swearing every night.

am going to assume that you have gone through all the other potential causes for sleepwalking (causing secondary sleepwalking, meaning the sleepwalking is actually being caused by some other identifiable disorder), and the underlying disorder has either been identified as not being present in your child, or it is present and remedied, yet still the sleepwalking persists. All other causes either accounted for or treated, sir!

So here is the full-treatment checklist:

☐ Sleep schedule is routine and structured seven days a week with an adequate amount of sleep opportunity and a comfortable sleeping environment (not too warm).*

☐ If there is a history of or evidence for GERD, consider a trial of anti-GERD medications.

☐ If the timing of events is relatively predictable, introducing a forced awakening fifteen minutes prior to the typical sleepwalking onset can be helpful. These awakenings should be done every night for a month.

☐ While no medications have been found effective for sleepwalking in clinical studies, some kids improve after taking gabapentin, longer-acting benzodiazepines, or tricyclic antidepressants before bedtime.

☐ For some children, counseling or presleep meditation/visualization can be helpful.

☐ If necessary, consider an overnight sleep study to evaluate the overnight sleep quality and to look for cues to what is triggering these behaviors.

Parasomnias Related to Eating

Another parasomnia variant found in children is nocturnal sleep-related eating disorder (NSRED). Children who struggle with NSRED often awaken from sleep to seek and consume food. In addition to the absence

---

* You know, the basics!

of memory for the event, the types of food and quantity of food consumed can be atypical.

NSRED can affect up to 5 percent of children in the general population, although numbers in young children are poorly reported and studied. It has been estimated that the number can more than triple in children and young adults with eating disorders. The use of some psychoactive medications in kids has been shown to cause nocturnal eating.

It is important to distinguish this disorder from nighttime eating syndrome (NES), in which the individual has full awareness of their eating. Despite the fact that NES happens at night, it is more often considered an eating disorder and not a parasomnia.

The treatment for NSRED is similar to that of sleepwalking, and many of the same treatments apply. While never studied in children, a drug called topiramate did show promise in a 2003 limited adult study. Given its frequent use in children for other purposes, this medication could be a consideration in difficult cases. The treatment of NSRED should also address ancillary effects of the disorder, such as significant weight gain by the child as well as a need to limit access to food, kitchen utensils, and appliances that could result in injury if carelessly operated. Locking cabinets or putting alarms on refrigerators can help to alert others that an episode is underway.

Other Movement Disorders Related to Sleep

It is worth noting that all the disorders described in this chapter represent complex movements that arise from sleep. Getting up and eating, jumping off a bed, and so on. Before we leave this chapter, I want to touch upon another group of nocturnal movements that tend to be much simpler but nevertheless are frequently misidentified as parasomnias.

These bedtime behaviors are often called sleep-related movement disorders. The most common of which is restless legs syndrome and the closely related periodic limb movement disorder, both of which we will cover in the next chapter. Other disorders in this group include teeth grinding (bruxism), leg cramps, and sleep-related rhythmic movement disorder.

Bruxism

Bruxism, or teeth grinding, is quite common in kids. Depending on the study and the criteria used to define bruxism, as many as 50 percent of kids grind or clench their jaw in some fashion during sleep. The condition tends to peak around ages five to seven, and the majority will eventually outgrow the condition. If the condition persists, it can cause significant problems, most notably teeth damage, jaw pain, and headache.

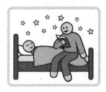 If your child has bruxism, it is important to contact a dentist immediately. It can often take time to determine the root cause of the bruxism, and in the meantime, your dentist will be able to help map out a plan for the protection of your child's teeth.

There are several conditions that may lead to bruxism:

- Does your child have a breathing disturbance at night, or has she been diagnosed with sleep apnea (see chapter 13)? If so, treating the disruptive breathing may immediately improve or eliminate the bruxism. While the weight of the scientific evidence linking sleep apnea treatment and bruxism in children is lacking, in adults, there seems to be a very strong correlation between the treatment of apnea and the resultant elimination of bruxism. The correlation in adults is so strong that it is debated whether bruxism truly exists during sleep but rather is always the result of some arousal from sleep . . . like, say, a breathing arousal. In one study, for example, sixty-seven episodes of bruxism were noted in untreated sleep apnea patients. All the events were eliminated with the addition of CPAP therapy.

- Anxiety has been linked to the occurrence of bruxism in pediatric studies. In a 2015 cross-sectional study, children with bruxism were scored higher by their parents on anxiety scales than children who did not exhibit bruxism.

- Insomnia is another common condition seen with bruxism. This makes sense if you consider the underlying role that anxiety plays in both. Treatment of the insomnia, anxiety, or ideally both can dramatically improve bruxism.

- Disorders of attention like ADHD can play a role in the development of bruxism in one of two ways. First, the disorder of ADHD itself is an independent risk factor for bruxism. Furthermore, bruxism is a common side effect of the medications typically used to treat ADHD.

- Finally, does your child show symptoms of gastroesophageal reflux? Studies have identified GERD as a risk factor for bruxism.

Sleep-Related Rhythmic Movement Disorder

This is one of the most interesting sleep disorders out there, because it is quite common, yet nobody ever talks about it because it is so bizarre.

A mother of a young boy was spending the night with him in a hotel room during a travel soccer event. As they were going to sleep, she heard a rhythmic sound coming from her son's bed. She initially (and embarrassingly) concluded that he was masturbating, despite the fact that she was less than ten feet away. "My husband and I often heard sounds coming from his bedroom that we thought best to ignore." As the movements intensified, she decided to turn on a light and see what was happening. "I was scared that he was going to injure himself. When I turned on my cell phone flashlight, he looked absolutely possessed. He was wildly flailing left and right in the bed, violently shaking his head as he aggressively flipped from his left side to right side in the bed.

Half unconscious, her son said, "What's wrong? Why are you shining that on me?"

"Sweetheart, you were rocking so hard back and forth, I thought something was wrong."

"What are you talking about?"

Rhythmic movements associated with sleep onset are common. These movements typically begin within the first one to two years of life, with the incidence precipitously declining with age. It is estimated that despite some form of rhythmic movement being present in 60 percent of nine-month-olds, the number drops to 5 percent by the time a child turns five.

These movements are most commonly associated with sleep onset, but in some cases, they can persist into the first part of the night. Because these actions happen on the brink of sleep, consciousness and awareness of the movements is variable, with most having no awareness of the events. Despite being a condition largely confined to the realm of children, I often see adults experiencing these movements in my clinic. I suspect that a combination of parental obliviousness and expectation that kids are restless when they sleep is to blame. Generally, when the condition persists to an older age, it is a romantic bed partner who usually sounds the alarm.

In my clinic, I have seen adult head bangers, thumb suckers, hair twirlers/pullers, as well as freestyle kickers. Vocalizations like humming can sometimes accompany the movements. The most common movements are whole-body rocking, head banging (typically in the prone position, the child will forcibly slam her head into a pillow or the mattress), or head rolling (in the supine position, the child will shake her head forcefully back and forth). In some cases, the movements will be combined.

And this is where the movement goes from just being a movement to being a disorder. Usually, the episodes of these movements are brief and harmless. Occasionally bouts are prolonged and result in injury. When the timing of the movements goes well past childhood, or injuries arise, it is typically labeled a disorder.

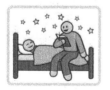 I was taught that a stereotyped movement or behavior at night was a seizure until proven otherwise. It is highly unlikely that your child's shaking before falling asleep at night is a seizure, but it is absolutely worth considering. Keep in mind that a seizure diagnosis is often the obvious diagnosis based upon the way it appears, but it can be

incorrect. Overnight sleep studies or inpatient EEG monitoring are useful in distinguishing the two disorders. A careful review of medications should be done as the condition can be linked to certain drugs. In some cases, the disorder can be linked to autism or other developmental disorders. The condition is thought to occasionally run in families and has even been reported in identical twins.

It is extremely important to make sure the bed and surrounding area are free from items that could lead to injury if struck. Add padding to headboards and bedside table edges to help reduce the risk of injury from rocking or head banging.

Pharmacological treatment, when needed, usually consists of medicating with benzodiazepines like clonazepam. In limited studies, these drugs demonstrated a mild reduction of symptoms via their calming effects on the central nervous system. There are older studies evaluating the use of "overpracticing" techniques as a general treatment for self-injurious behaviors. These therapies stress the child repeating or practicing the behaviors while fully awake and conscious in an effort to create awareness and control.

 Jamie came to my clinic soon after her nocturnal joyride. Her concerned mother made the trek to come with her. A careful history revealed a driven young woman who often did not get adequate or consistent sleep. When she did have the opportunity to sleep, she often took Ambien, "so that the sleep I get is as good as it can be."

By discontinuing the Ambien and working harder to ensure a more appropriate sleep schedule, Jamie's behaviors dramatically lessened and no further treatment was required.

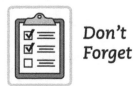

Don't Forget

1. Parasomnias are common and do not necessarily require treatment.

2. Ensuring the safety of the child is often the first and primary concern.

3. These disorders often are the result of underlying medication side effects and other disorders.

11

Restless Legs Syndrome/Periodic Limb Movement Disorder

"If You Can't Sit Still During My Class, You Can Fidget Out in the Hall."

 Colby is a twelve-year-old boy who was referred to my office because of "academic and behavioral decline" as well as occasional bed-wetting, just frequent enough to be a concern. He is a robust boy who enjoys football and school, and he is a good student.

"Ever since we can remember, Colby has struggled with his sleep," his father reports. He paints a picture of a completely dismantled bed every morning. "I understand how a bed might be a little messy in the morning, but Colby destroys his bed. He's completely untucked the sheet, wadded it up, and is using it as a pillow because his real pillow is on the other side of the room. The bottom sheet and mattress pad are half pulled off, and the mattress itself is exposed. Colby is often turned sideways or a whole 180 degrees. When the sheet manages to stay on, he wears holes in it where his feet have repeatedly rubbed it threadbare."

Outside of looking tired (and actually napping during the visit), he seems perfectly normal. The emergence of his school problems has coincided with sleep issues, which have been chalked up to anxiety and possible inattentiveness. Strangely, despite difficulties sleeping at night, he has absolutely no trouble falling asleep at other times of the day, including at school. Hot baths and a weighted blanket recommended by a friend have been helpful, but what really helps Colby sleep is for Mom to rub his legs, which are often affected by growing pains.

Colby's mom rolls her eyes and elaborates with a sigh. "I wouldn't mind rubbing his legs so much if I didn't have to do it for his brother and father every night too!"

~ ~ ~

Chances are, if you ask parents and pediatricians alike to compile a list of common sleep disorders seen in kids under the age of twenty-one, one of the most common disorders would not make the list at all. What's more unusual is that 25 percent of individuals with the condition report that it started in childhood, between the ages of ten and twenty.

What Is Restless Legs Syndrome?

The condition I'm talking about is restless legs syndrome (RLS), and I fudged a little when I said it was common. It's definitely common in the adult population, and while I suspect it's pretty common in the pediatric population, up until recently, the incidence in kids was largely unknown. Brand-new research has begun to shed a light on this disorder, determining that 8.6 percent of children may be at risk for developing RLS, with that incidence jumping up to 13 percent in kids who have at least one parent with RLS.

 RLS is a neurologic disorder first described in medical literature by Thomas Willis in 1672.* Willis was a pioneering English physician who wrote in his ambitiously titled book *Two Discourses Concerning the Soul of Brutes, Which Is that of*

---

* This was just shy of two hundred years before our friend Anna Steese Richardson's birth, in 1865.

the Vital and Sensitive of Man that certain psychiatric conditions could be treated by being beaten about with sticks. When it comes to doctors of the 1600s, you win some (discovered RLS!) and you lose some (*How will you ever improve the hysteria creeping upon your child when he sleepeth if you do not permit me to beat the nervous liquor from the pores of his brain with my stick?*). Medicinal stick beatings fortunately never caught on and disappeared along with Willis's RLS discovery until 1945, when the term "restless legs" was coined by Swedish neurologist and pioneer of the hyphenated first name Karl-Axel Ekbom.* In his description of the disorder, he wrote about "growing pains" and theorized that these were a similar but separate disorder seen only in childhood. Several years later, the symptom of growing pains was linked to a higher likelihood that an individual would develop restless legs syndrome later in life. With time, genetic underpinnings of the disorder were worked out after observations of the disorder were clearly seen running through families.

Symptoms of Restless Legs Syndrome

So let's get down to what this disorder entails. If you look up the definition, you will see something like this:

> *RLS is a sensory and motor disorder characterized by an uncontrollable sensation in the legs accompanied by an irresistible urge to move the legs, which usually results in partial or complete resolution immediately albeit transiently.*

The truth of the matter: restless legs is a very hard disorder to describe . . . even for people like me who have it.† It is a damn strange feeling. Does it hurt? No. Is it like a cramp? Uh, not really but . . . Is it

---

* For reasons unclear to me, perhaps to make people take this condition more seriously, there is a push to rename restless legs syndrome Willis Ekbom disease. Notice how this wonderfully descriptive name rolls effortlessly off the tongue.

† I have had RLS sporadically for years. I remember as a child feeling an irresistible urge to get on the floor of the family room while I was watching *The A-Team* and

achy? No, but you are getting warmer. While the condition is often de-scribed as a crawling feeling, like you have earthworms in your legs, I'm not sure that captures the essence of the feeling. Think of the sensation of feeling an itch that you are not allowed to scratch. Now, instead of the superficial prickliness you feel on your skin, submerge that feeling deep into the muscles of your legs. And instead of a prickly feeling, turn down the treble and turn up the bass of that discomfort. Maybe that paints a picture of how it feels.

I can imagine you reading that description and saying, *Turn up the bass . . . What in the world is he talking about?* I can't easily answer that question, but just think that if a reasonably educated person like me whose mother was an English teacher can only express himself like that, think of how hard it is for a child to describe the problem . . . or frankly even recognize the disorder as a problem. This is why RLS is so underdi-agnosed in children. The simple fact is that there is extreme difficulty in communicating the problem, and the pediatrician/primary care doctor (with whom they will be interacting), often does not have the knowledge of the condition to accurately detect and diagnose it.

So RLS is an uncomfortable feeling your child has in the evening be-fore he goes to bed. Who cares? It is an internal tickle when he's awake. What's the big deal? The big deal is that RLS is often associated with a condition called periodic limb movement disorder (PLMD). As the name implies, kids who also have PLMD periodically move their legs at night.* While it is often described as a kick, it is typically far more subtle than the word "kick" implies. Think of it as a twitch, a single toe tap, or a brief scissoring motion of the legs as a child lies on his side.

For the most part, legs (or any other body part) don't move without

---

doing a body movement I can only describe as making a snow angel to make my legs feel better.

* And by periodically, I mean an observant parent could literally predict to the sec-ond when their sleeping child's leg will kick: Kick . . . Seventeen seconds . . . Kick . . . Seventeen seconds . . . Kick . . . etc.

the brain's authorization, so as you watch these leg movements happen, think about what is really going on here:

1. Child goes to sleep (no thanks to the RLS, which can make that act difficult because of the discomfort they feel while awake and trying to sleep).

2. Once asleep, the child's legs move because the brain/PLMD causes them to do so.

3. This creates an arousal or awakening in the child.

4. The leg movement ends, and the child falls back to sleep (usually, but again, sometimes the RLS makes this difficult).

5. Repeat the process hundreds of times during the night.

Pay particular attention to item #3. Basically, it says the child wakes up. In fact, the child wakes up a ton. Now, think way back to the first chapter of this book and how we all strive for a continuous, deep, robust sleep. Reconcile that utopian sleep with your child who awakens every seventeen seconds to move his legs. This is the devil in the disease. Are the leg movements dangerous, concerning, or problematic in and of themselves? No. In fact I have fretted over treating these nocturnal movements in some kids because I worry that I may be eliminating their sole source of exercise. The danger is in the sleep disturbance and the complete disruption to the overall flow of sleep.

To summarize quickly, RLS is a disruptive feeling of discomfort your child may feel while awake that can inhibit their ability to relax and easily fall asleep. In approximately 70 percent of kids with RLS, they will also exhibit PLMD during sleep. Unlike the restlessness they experience at night, individuals are often not aware of the periodic limb movements.

A certain amount of restlessness and movement is perfectly normal and acceptable in children. When you have been around kids and parents of kids with this condition, you quickly see that their kid's movements are on a whole new level. The destruction of the bed (and sometimes the bed linens) as mentioned earlier is pretty common. Unlike most kids who have the same *Star Wars* sheets on their bed for their entire childhood (and beyond*), the idea that these kids could use the same sheets for more than a year or two is crazy because of how much they abuse them.

Beyond the linens catastrophe, there can be more severe situations of room destruction. One teenage patient said he shook his leg so violently that he would inadvertently kick the wall and damage the drywall. Another teen kicked so frequently and violently that his bed would shift across the floor during the night and end up in a different place the following morning.

The most common complaint about a child with RLS/PLMD relates to the hotel stay. Sleeping in more confined quarters is not fun under these circumstances. In these situations, there is a kind of bed lottery that happens. In families who have a child with RLS/PLMD, nobody wants to draw the short straw and have to sleep with her. Family members will tell stories about the time Mom had to share a bed with the affected child, and how eventually Mom was forced to get out of bed and sleep in the bathtub. This is often the way the problem comes to the attention of a family member and eventually a physician.

Another aspect of Colby's story that is very commonly seen in RLS is the ongoing trouble with growing pains. They often have unusual rituals that accompany sleep. Mom or Dad rubbing their legs is certainly a common characteristic. Weight on their legs is another. Sometimes they sleep under heavy blankets, often folded up to just compress their legs. Weighted blankets, which have come into fashion more recently, can provide these kids a sense of relief. Occasionally, affected youths will develop unusual exercise rituals to try to "work the feelings out" before bed. Finally, some find that hot baths, or even use of a hot tub is key to getting the symptoms to go away.

Finally, Colby's mom makes a comment that seems to insinuate that other people in the family have the problem. Diagnostically, this can be

---

* It's humbling to come home for college winter break and sleep in a twin bed made up with Yoda sheets.

a blessing or a curse. It is a blessing if a parent has been diagnosed and she can make the diagnosis herself by recognizing the shared symptoms. The curse occurs when family members have the condition, but have never been diagnosed. In these cases, what they observe in their children is mistakenly seen as normal for everyone because it is the norm for the family.

Diagnosing Restless Legs Syndrome

A diagnosis can be made with the help of a solid clinical history coupled with the existence of many features consistent with RLS. Generally, the diagnosis of RLS is a clinical diagnosis, which means that no blood tests or imaging studies are necessary. It is just a clinician listening carefully to the parents' and the kid's story and seeing if the following criteria are met. While the adult and pediatric criteria are largely the same, language, intellect, and parental reporting is factored into the equation when it comes to diagnosing a child with RLS:

- Is your child displaying restlessness or uneasiness?

- Does the problem seem to be worse in the evening and better during the day?

- Does inactivity make the condition worse?

- Does movement or exercise seem to make it better or relieve the feeling all together?

It's important that the condition be described in the child's own words and that other causes of discomfort, such as itching/dermatitis, strains, positional numbness (legs falling asleep), are ruled out.

As you can imagine, these questions are a little tougher for a child to answer than "Does your throat hurt when you swallow?" or "Did your brother stick a bead up your nose?" Depending on the situation, it may be helpful to perform a sleep study on the child to help support the diagnosis and to rule out other conditions that might be affecting sleep.

The Consequences of RLS

Now that you've established a diagnosis of RLS and you know that your child is awakening up to hundreds of times a night due to this disorder, it's time to assess the damage that RLS causes. Aside from producing an incredibly cranky kid, children with RLS experience all kinds of issues stemming from their sleep. Because of the disruption in rest, RLS primarily causes excessive daytime sleepiness. With the near constant leg movements, the disorder can present as insomnia or a significant difficulty with maintaining sleep during the night (primarily the first half of the night when the periodic movements tend to be the worst). In kids, if you disrupt sleep, you are invariably going to get attention issues, problems with behavior, conduct, and irritability and inattentiveness presenting like ADHD. How many kids do you know who are treated for ADHD? How many kids do you know who are treated for RLS? Yep . . . it is a problem!

Treatment of RLS in Children

This is a tough one. I've given you all of this lead-up just so I can tell you that sleep specialists really can't agree on this item. As of the writing of this book, there are as many quality randomized studies showing that using a ThighMaster for twenty minutes within thirty to sixty minutes of bedtime is as effective at treating RLS as any other medication you can name, including the drugs we use for adults. Even the American Academy of Sleep Medicine has not listed treatments they consider approved.

Treatment should always start by ensuring adequate sleep and good sleep scheduling, as consistent sleep schedules can improve symptoms. Evaluate your child's concurrent medications, as some antidepressants or mood-altering agents (e.g., lithium) can worsen symptoms. Because the disorder is linked to dopamine, drugs like prochlorperazine and metoclopramide that block dopamine might cause the problem or make it worse. Activity level is an unusual variable, with some children responding positively to exercise or stretching before bed, while others report symptom exacerbation. Heavy food intake prior to sleep, as well as chocolate, tea, caffeine, or nitrates can cause inflammation and make RLS symptoms worse.

Finally, it may be worth exploring your child's thyroid status, kidney health, and ferritin (iron) level during their medical workup. Chronic renal insufficiency, hypothyroidism, and low ferritin have been linked to increased incidence of RLS. While these causes and treatments have not been studied extensively in children, they are known precipitants in adults.

Restless Sleep Disorder

This disorder was only recently discovered and characterized by a group led by Dr. Lourdes DelRosso, a sleep expert and pulmonologist at the University of Washington School of Medicine and Seattle Children's Hospital. The disorder is found in an estimated 7 percent of children ages six to eighteen.

The symptoms of the condition involve large body movements during sleep that are not confined to the legs. They occur at least five times an hour, at least three times a week for three months. Perhaps most important, the movements result in excessive daytime sleepiness and other significant functional impairments. As in RLS, treatment with iron may help improve symptoms.

 Colby ended up being what we call a "three for the price of one" or sometimes a "family discount." What that means is one patient gets treated, and soon after, other members of his family get treated as well. In this case it was brother and father. Because of his larger size and snoring, Colby ended up having a sleep study. The bed-wetting history was considered as well.

Here is a segment of his sleep study.

Let's quickly orient ourselves to what we are looking at. This is a slightly different sleep study than you are used to in this book. Most of the previous sleep study samples show a total of thirty seconds of sleep recording from left to right (one epoch). In this view, we have compressed the window so that now, from the left side of the segment to the right is

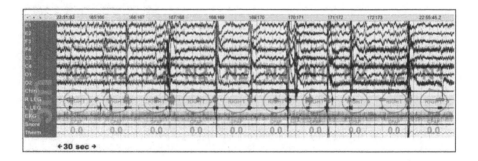

actually five minutes or ten epochs. You can see the ten sections of thirty seconds divided by the thin vertical lines. Sleep doctors often compress studies like this if they are trying to see trends occurring over a long period of time. Notice how this view is not great for trends occurring over a short period when looking for things like heart rate, for instance.

What you are seeing in this segment is a child who demonstrates approximately seventeen discreet movements of his legs within ten minutes. Those movements are indicated by the bursts of activity measured by the electrode on his right leg (R LEG). That's not the troubling part. The worst part is the fact that if you look up from the leg movements, there are a series of vertical disruptions in the relatively peaceful background waves of his sleep. Ten minutes of sleep. Seventeen episodes of essentially being jerked awake by leg movements. No wonder Colby was struggling.

The story had a fantastic ending. After ensuring sleep quality and quantity was top shelf and checking the family's ferritin levels (all well above normal*), we started Colby on a small dose of ropinirole taken thirty minutes before bedtime, and his symptoms resolved almost immediately, as did his brother's and father's.

* Values >7 ng/mL are often reported as normal ferritin levels in children. While there is no research in children, research in adults indicates that levels greater than 50–100 ng/ml are more ideal for those with RLS. Supplemental iron can be helpful for some adults with low ferritin and RLS.

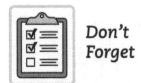 **Don't Forget**

1. Restless legs syndrome is a common and highly disruptive sleep disorder that can look like insomnia and other sleep complaints.

2. Most children with RLS will have accompanying periodic limb movement disorder.

3. RLS/PLMD is highly hereditary and treatable if the disorder is recognized.

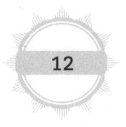

12

Enuresis

Despite What Your Pediatrician Keeps Telling You, This Is Not Normal!

 There is something unique and heartbreaking about a clinic visit regarding enuresis—the involuntary discharge of urine—in a child. In my experience, the child always comes with Mom only. For many of the kids who visit my office, there is a certain obliviousness about them in the exam room. They don't really seem to know why they are in my office; in some cases, they look surprised that the visit is regarding them. This is not the case for the child with enuresis. They know who the visit is for and are painfully aware of why they are there. This was absolutely the case for Stuart.

Stuart is a small eleven-year-old boy who is totally engaged from the start.

"Good morning. You must be Stuart. I'm Chris. What can I do for you?"

"I always wet the bed, and my doctor said it might be because of my sleep." Stuart is taken care of by a total kick-ass pediatrician in my region who is always on top of the sleep of her patients. She often refers children to me who she thinks need to be evaluated for attention issues, behavioral issues, sleepiness issues, and yes, enuresis issues.

I put on my best engaged but unimpressed face. "Okay. Lots of kids and adults come to this clinic because they wet the bed at night. You have no idea how common it is. I know it is not a fun thing to talk about, but it is no big deal. We see college students sometimes who wet the bed. We are going to figure out how we can get it taken care of, okay?" To me, the most important thing to do in the moment is to make sure that when Stuart leaves the clinic, he does not feel like some freak. My demeanor and tone are meant to convey confidence and experience, but above everything else, comfort. This is an annoying and inconvenient problem that is solvable and will get better. Nothing more.

As Stuart gives me his history, it is clear that the issue is quite socially disruptive. He has basically one friend he feels comfortable having over for sleepovers. No sharing hotel rooms with others. No sleeping bags or camping. No staying at others' homes.

That alone is a tough spot to be in. His stature was another. When asked, "How does your size compare to the other boys in the class?" his response is a timid, "I'm the second smallest." Given his first name, you can imagine the natural nickname. At his last pediatrician's visit, he was about four foot five (fifty-three inches), about three inches shorter than the average eleven-year-old. What was more concerning was that his growth seemed to be "falling off the curve." In other words, in the years prior, he was not exactly tall for his age, but until age eight, he was at least at the average height for a boy his age. According to Mom, this time period corresponded to the reappearance of his bed-wetting.

"What do you mean by reappearance? Was Stuart dry for a period of time and then went back to bed-wetting?"

"Yes," his mother replies. "We thought it was related to school stress because Stuart had a difficult third-grade experience and things at home were stressful for a period of time. When those things 'stabilized,' the bed-wetting did not. In fact, it seemed to worsen."*

---

* "Stabilized" referred to academic and attention issues at school. Some acting out and mild oppositional defiance. While there was some talk of ADHD evaluation, it

Otherwise, Stuart is a healthy boy. As far as interventions that have been tried, Stuart was put on desmopressin (DDAVP*), an antidiuretic, with limited improvement. Fluid restriction proved to be ineffective. An enuresis alarm was utilized for about a week, but abandoned because of "stressing out my husband and scaring Stuart's little brother [in the same bedroom] every night. It's just not worth it."

When we discuss Stuart's sleep, he is described as restless and often complaining of being tired. He has no history of snoring or breathing disturbances at night.

~ ~ ~

Children go to the bathroom. From what I have read, adults do as well. There, we are talking about pee. I thought bringing the subject up would be awkward, but it really feels good to have the topic just out there.

For many parents, bed-wetting is not just an issue with babies. These issues can persist deep into childhood or reappear after disappearing for some time. Often, this problem can have its roots in sleep. Unfortunately, these conditions are often inappropriately ignored or incorrectly treated by primary care physicians, and the consequences are not trivial. In a 2016 study on enuresis, all eighty-seven children who were subjects in the study were punished in some way by their parents. Nearly half the kids who had parents who struggled with enuresis themselves as children were physically punished.

Let's start with some definitions.

Enuresis is simply involuntary urination. No specific population or age group is implied, nor is a specific time of day designated. When

---

never panned out, and with some limited counseling, teacher intervention, and adjustment of Stuart's school schedule, things improved.

* DDAVP (which stands for 1-deamino-8-D-arginine vasopressin) is a synthetic chemical similar to arginine vasopressin, which is released from the brain's pituitary gland during times when the body is low on volume, causing the body to hang on to urine. Interestingly, arginine vasopressin also plays a role in coagulation, with the drug serving as an essential treatment for various clotting disorders.

exploring enuresis in this book, we are talking primarily about pediatric nocturnal enuresis . . . children wetting the bed at night. Keep in mind, this is different than nocturia, which is simply waking up and going to the bathroom at night.

 The views on enuresis have changed a lot over the years. In the dark ages, I'm sure it was a sign your child was possessed and needed to be cast into a nearby well. Even in the early 1900s, it was virtually always chalked up to psychiatric issues or problems with parenting, which just meant the parents were cast into the well instead.

Turning to our resident expert on children of yesteryear, Anna Steese Richardson had some pretty lofty expectations of children and their mothers at the turn of the twentieth century. Her advice firmly informed parents that by two years of age, the child, "should be completely broken of the habit." Ouch. I wouldn't want to show my face at the local church ladies' social with a three-year-old child still wetting the bed.

If the child did not have themselves together by age two, it was recommended that they be put on a little training "chamber" every hour on the hour the entire day *and night*, with the intervals lengthened by thirty minutes at two- to three-week intervals. Yowza! As someone who sometimes struggles to make sure his kids take their antibiotics twice a day for ten days, this seems like a pretty huge ask of a mother! Fortunately, it is pretty much guaranteed to work by the time your child is six. The devastation brought upon Mom's sleep must have been covered in a later publication.

For the stubborn child for whom the *Harry Potty and the Chamber of Secrets* method was ineffective, the treatment became quite severe—the dry evening meal. I imagine you can guess what this entailed. Virtually no liquids or moist foods after 4:00 p.m. Exceptions: butter may be served with dry cereal, applesauce may be used to "moisten" bread or crackers, and under no circumstance should a child be given coffee or tea, as these are not "juvenile beverages."

If these actions do not work, Richardson concludes her enuresis advice with a clear message: "If the habit has grown upon the child, discipline alone will cure it."*

What Is Nocturnal Enuresis?

In our enlightened times, it has become abundantly clear that nocturnal enuresis can have multiple causes that relate to anatomical and urological conditions, medication side effects, and, yes, sleep disorders, primarily conditions that increase arousals from sleep. Today, before jumping right to concluding there is something wrong with a child's brain or psyche, there are multiple boxes to check in the enuresis workup.

One stop on the checklist in recent years has been the sleep specialist. Here, the kid is evaluated for conditions affecting sleep that might lead to enuresis. To me, the action is a no-brainer, as there is little risk involved in the whole affair and potentially some high reward (which absolutely makes my day).

To get started, I think it is very important for parents to have an understanding of what is considered normal in terms of potty training, nocturnal bladder control, and bed-wetting in children and what would be considered exceptional.† Currently, multiple epidemiological studies have concluded that enuresis continues to be present in about 15 to 25 percent of five-year-old children. In a preschool class of twenty-five five-year-olds, five kids are still wetting the bed. Overall, for kids in the six-to-twelve age range, the percentage of kids with enuresis is somewhere between 1.4 and 28 percent.

Studies like this have led to the generally agreed upon age of five as being the birthday after which we no longer consider bed-wetting to be a normal occurrence. Generally, two or more episodes/month is considered the cutoff. The time between five and seven years old is a bit hazy,

---

* So while it is not overtly spelled out, I take this to mean putting a child on the chamber every hour and mercilessly hitting him with a switch on the half hour if no pee-pees have been produced. All other household chores should be worked into the intervening times. Easy.

† And by the way, your child is exceptional even if he wets the bed every night!

but after five, most experts agree it is time to talk to someone, and I think so too. Is it true that some bed-wetting will subside on its own after age seven? Absolutely. As many as 15 percent of children per year will shake the problem. Still, for the 85 percent not making the cut every year, it is having a tremendous effect on their psyche—no sleepovers, no summer camps, no big-girl underwear at night.

Like sleepwalking, there is a big genetic component, with multiple genes being related to the emergence of enuresis. It is estimated that around 30 percent of children who struggle with enuresis are genetically inclined to have the problem. In one study, 65 percent of children with nocturnal enuresis had a family member who experienced the same problem.

So what might children be inheriting? What are the various causes of pediatric enuresis? These diverse mechanisms are on full display in one Italian study of four hundred children ages five to sixteen (with approximately a three-to-one boy-to-girl ratio). In the study, 31.2 percent of cases seemed to have a hereditary component, but a full two-thirds of the cases were something else. Among the common causes found were:

urogenital abnormalities (15.7 percent);
constipation (14.5 percent);
cardiovascular/innocent heart murmur (21.4 percent);
snoring/breathing disturbance (13.7 percent);
restless sleep (5.7 percent);
somniloquy (23.7 percent);
bruxism (14.7 percent);
medications (e.g., valproate).

The point to be made here is that even though enuresis can be an inherited condition that will disappear over time, that is not always correct. If we are putting all the causes of enuresis on the table, the "one day, like a miracle, it will disappear" strategy is really missing the target.

In looking at the aforementioned list of causes, we can largely group the origins of enuresis into three main categories.

1. Anatomical abnormalities (e.g., urogenital abnormalities).

2. Overproduction of urine (polyuria), particularly at night.

3. Sleep disturbances (e.g., restless sleep, snoring, etc.).

Anatomical Abnormalities

I'm largely going to leave the anatomical abnormalities to the urologists, who are the experts. Generally, just think of these causes as being related to the mechanics of voiding not working properly. For example, when we urinate, our detrusor muscle contracts and our urinary sphincter muscle relaxes, causing voiding of the bladder. In babies, this entire process is a reflex, stimulated by the stretch of the bladder as it fills. As children mature, we gain voluntary control over the relaxation of the sphincter muscle, allowing us significant control over when we void. This control can be overridden if the production of urine is high and the bladder is overfilled, thus triggering the response. We have all seen this in the child who tried to hold it until the next rest stop but ultimately failed.

Sometimes, enuresis can be caused by anatomical abnormalities or dysfunctions. Urologists are able to evaluate and test children to make sure these parts and processes are working properly. They can also evaluate chronic urinary tract infections as a cause for enuresis. A visit to a urologist is usually one of the first stops for a child with problematic enuresis.

Overproduction of Urine

A logical theory about enuresis has been that the child has consumed too much fluid and therefore needs to have their intake reduced or restricted to keep them dry at night. Seems logical. Got a leaky pipe? Shutting off the water to the house should do the trick. This theory was popular in the 1980s, when research began to point to polyuria, the overproduction of urine, as a cause of nocturnal enuresis. This ushered in a more scientifically rigorous approach to enuresis and helped marginalize theories that it was purely a psychological phenomenon. Until recently, this was a widely held theory with many enuresis treatments geared toward reducing the production of urine. Interventions could be as simple as limiting fluid intake to giving medications like desmopressin (DDAVP), an antidiuretic, to reduce the urge to urinate.*

Over time, the polyuria theory has come into question. Why do many kids with polyuria not have enuresis? Why do the kids with enuresis not awaken when the bed-wetting happens? Recently, research centering around these questions suggests that the overproduction of urine may be the *result* of other causes of enuresis (like sleep-related enuresis), rather than the cause.

This leads us to another enuresis mechanism: disorders of sleep and arousal. After your kid's pipes and pumps have been determined to be in the right place and working properly, it is time to focus on sleep. Sleep disturbances are often found in children with enuresis.

Sleep Disturbances

Anyone who has ever been in a situation where urination needs to happen but it was impossible to do so knows that the feeling can be overwhelming. I personally remember walking back to my hotel from a meeting in Manhattan and suddenly having the urge come upon me. There was no easy place to duck into, and the urge quickly became all-encompassing. By the time I decided to duck into a fancy hotel and pretend that I was staying there, the pain was overwhelming, and I actually felt like my bladder was going to explode and my kidneys were going to rupture from the backflow of urine building inside of me. As I came upon the restroom off the lobby, I had decided that if the door to the lobby was locked, I was going to relieve myself in a nearby plant. Mercifully, it was unlocked. As I urinated, the feeling was so intense that I literally started to develop tunnel vision and thought I might black out. I held it together and tried to casually walk out of the hotel.

I share this personal story to illustrate a simple fact: the urge to urinate is a strong one. Very strong. Given that the stretching of the bladder and the contraction of the detrusor muscle produce very strong sensations,

---

* I have to say that limiting a child's fluid intake to help with bed-wetting has never made sense to me. It is like finding an oil leak in your car and your mechanic suggesting limiting the oil you put into your automobile as a solution.

what do you think about the depth of sleep in a child who can sleep through it all (not to mention the sensation of suddenly being wet)?

Here, we start to touch upon the concept of light or deep sleepers. Understanding that the terms "light sleep" and "deep sleep" can refer to specific sleep stages as we discussed in chapter 2, these terms are more commonly used to describe children who are easily awakened from sleep ("light sleepers") or those who are not ("deep sleepers"). To avoid confusion, a better way to think about this concept is using the term "arousal threshold." An arousal threshold is the strength of a stimulus necessary to produce an arousal from sleep. Therefore, light sleepers have a low arousal threshold and deep sleepers a high arousal threshold.* In children with enuresis, it has been shown that their general arousal thresholds are higher, giving them the ability to sleep through the typically awakening stimuli of having to urinate.

Wow, sleep so deep you can sleep through the painful expansion of your bladder. That must be some outrageously good sleep, right? Sleep so deep we can't even wake her up in the morning. She must be a champion when it comes to sleep. Isn't sleeping deeply what every person in a sleeping pill commercial is after?

Here again we can see the difference between healthy sleep, deep sleep as measured on a sleep study, and a "deep-sleeping" child. In 2009, a study of twenty-nine boys and girls ages five to nineteen with diagnosed enuresis was conducted to investigate the relationship between bed-wetting and sleep quality. The study demonstrated an exceptionally high percentage of children with periodic limb movements during the night. Despite the "deep sleep" of enuretic children, their sleep quality may be fragmented, poor, and marked by restlessness, abnormal amounts of movement, and other quality disruptors. Don't assume that children

---

* In general, the arousal threshold in deep sleep is higher than the arousal threshold in light sleep, so the terms are not altogether incorrect. It is important to recognize that differing arousal thresholds are not typically distinguishable via polysomnographic sleep studies. In other words, it is not possible to reliably distinguish high-threshold sleepers from low-threshold sleepers via a sleep study.

with enuresis are at least getting quality sleep—in many cases, they are not.

Traditional Treatments for Nocturnal Enuresis

The treatment of enuresis has a rich history that is well worth exploring. These treatments are perfectly valid and helpful in many situations. If your child is struggling with getting through the night dry, you may be familiar with some or all of them. Having a clear understanding of these methods may not only make you better equipped to deal with your child's bed-wetting but may also help convince doctors and insurance companies that a sleep study is necessary for your child's complete enuresis workup.

Behavioral Therapy

Multiple studies have concluded that behavioral therapy using some form of bed-wetting alarm is by far the most effective treatment for nocturnal enuresis. When compared to other therapies, the 75 percent success rate is much higher and the relapse rate is low. The downside to these therapies is that it can be quite traumatic to the child and family to be jolted awake every night by the buzzer that detects urine. Given that these devices can take upward of ten weeks to work, it should not be a surprise that the dropout rate is high. When I have helped patients and their families maximize the benefit of enuresis alarms, it is truly an all-hands-on-deck situation. For these alarms to work, there needs to be a substantial buy-in from the parents (I say parents and not parent because it probably takes two people coordinating their efforts for this to work).

A quick description of enuresis alarms: they are typically a pad that is placed underneath your sleeping child at night. The pad has a sensor in it that can detect minuscule amounts of water. When the pad detects said water, an extremely loud alarm is triggered, jolting your child and anyone within a three–city block radius awake. Ideally, your little one awakens, waddles off to the bathroom, finishes in the toilet what was started in the bed, and goes back to sleep without any further intervention from you.

This is not going to happen.

Remember the theories about enuretic children sleeping deeper and having higher arousal thresholds than normal children? Well, be prepared to be absolutely flabbergasted that your child has the superhero-like ability to sleep through an air-raid siren. I have been told by countless parents that they are more distressed by their child sleeping through the alarm than they are by the bed-wetting!

There are many things that need to happen with enuresis alarms, and you cannot simply rely upon your child to accomplish them on his own. First, you must ensure that your child gets up, out of bed, and finishes using the bathroom in the potty. For this reason, speed matters, because the quicker you can get to your child's room and help him get out of bed and to the toilet, the more likely he's going to have some urine left to void once he gets there. The completion of the act in the appropriate place (the bathroom) is very important for the treatment to work, and after a night or two, it is usually where things break down. Additionally, your child may also need some help cleaning the bed and resetting the alarm.*

Medications
Other therapies for enuresis can involve medications that may be useful for children who make too much urine (polyuria). Desmopressin (DDAVP) is commonly used to help reduce urinary volumes at night and lessen the pressure within the bladder.

Imipramine is another drug that is often used for nocturnal enuresis. Nobody knows why it works exactly. Its anticholinergic effects might reduce bladder contractibility (which is why its anticholinergic toxicity/ side effects can include urinary retention).† Who knows? It is really

---

* It might be helpful to put up a sign that reads, "75 percent" as in there is a 75 percent chance this goddamn alarm is going to work and help my child get through the night dry. You may need the encouragement heading into week six.

† Imipramine is a magical drug in neurology because it is used to treat just about everything. The drug is a tricyclic antidepressant, so its FDA approval is for depression. Off-label, it is used to treat enuresis, sleep paralysis, night terrors, nightmare disorder, sleepwalking, migraines, eating disorders, and panic disorders. I guess what I'm saying is, maybe talk to your doctor about trying imipramine for your kid.

the closest thing we have in sleep medicine to a "magic potion." In a 2019 study of forty children ages five to twelve, 83.3 percent of the kids getting imipramine showed significant improvement versus only 29.4 percent in the control group.

Fluid Restriction

Finally, we get to fluid restriction as a treatment for nocturnal enuresis.

Sigh.

Let's be frank. Is there any difference between fluid restriction as a therapy for your child's bed-wetting and starving your child who is struggling with obesity? I'm sorry, but it just sounds dumb at best and unhealthy at worst. Theories regarding enuretic children suggest that not only should fluids be unrestricted but also that some children with enuresis do not drink enough fluids. In fact, fluid restriction often results in an overcompensation of fluid intake at other times. At best, the division of fluid intake to 40 percent in the morning, 40 percent in the afternoon, and 20 percent in the evening can be considered. Evidence that fluid restriction works is minimal.

Anecdotally, there are reports of hypnosis and acupuncture treating enuresis in some less recent studies. I suspect that if you tell children that they have to see a "person who pokes you with needles to help with your bed-wetting," the mere suggestion would cure a significant number of cases! At this point, there are no large-scale studies proving their efficacy, but smaller older studies do exist. One study from 1985 showed hypnosis improved symptoms in a study of forty-eight eight- to thirteen-year-old boys, and it only took six months!

Sleep Evaluation/Treatment in Enuresis

The take-home message from this chapter is that once you have determined that your child might have issues with enuresis, it is time to act. You've spoken to your pediatrician. You have at least talked about a urological evaluation for your child. Maybe you have tried some pills and an alarm.

One intervention that may not be mentioned to you is a sleep evaluation. Nearly all the topics covered in this book that disturb sleep can be potential causes for enuresis, so it is very important to carefully monitor your child's sleep as a potential cause of enuresis. This consideration should involve, at a minimum, a very deep dive into the sleeping characteristics and habits of your child. I think an overnight in-lab sleep study is always a very reasonable age-appropriate evaluation tool.*

If a sleep study is performed, there are many disorders to screen for, and these disorders should be discussed prior to the study. It is absolutely fair to make sure that your sleep specialist is casting a wide net for these causative disorders. None are more important than sleep apnea, a very common cause of enuresis in children. In a 2012 study, fourteen previous studies were reviewed, looking at the association between sleep apnea and enuresis. Out of 3,550 children ages eighteen months to nineteen years with confirmed sleep apnea, nearly one-third also had enuresis. In these children, the repeated breathing disturbances provides the sleep fragmentation and frequent arousals that produce the sleepiness seen in these kids. Once again, we have the "deep" but "poor" sleeper who is the perfect candidate for enuresis.

In the same retrospective review study, the incidence of enuresis in children scheduled to undergo tonsillectomy was 31 percent (roughly the rate cited in the previous paragraph). Analysis of surgical outcomes revealed the postoperative rate of enuresis to be 16 percent. Surgery improved nearly 50 percent of enuresis seen in these children. In my clinic, I have seen repeated cases of tonsillectomies that led to immediate cessation of both snoring/sleep apnea as well as bed-wetting.

New research has also noticed a relationship between enuresis and restless legs syndrome in children. In a 2014 study, children with nocturnal enuresis showed a much higher incidence of periodic limb movements than children who were not restless at night. It is likely that the RLS is causing the enuresis.

---

* I often joke that the worst-case scenario with a sleep study is that it will be normal!

Nocturnal Emission

I told you we would talk about wet dreams a long time ago, and here we are. I feel that if we are writing a book about kids and sleep, it needs to at least be mentioned.

Nocturnal orgasms (sometimes referred to as nightfalls*) are common in adolescent sleepers and can happen in both boys and girls after puberty. With changing hormone levels, nocturnal emissions can become frequent occurrences in some boys. Eighty-three percent of boys will have at least one nocturnal emission in their lifetime, with an average frequency of approximately once every three weeks according to Kinsey's landmark studies.

 Stuart eventually underwent a sleep study. He and his father (!) spent a relatively uneventful night at the sleep center. His sleep study demonstrated the presence of sleep apnea that was quite significant for his age group (he averaged approximately twenty-one breathing disturbances/hour). After discussing the results of the study and available treatment options, his family elected for Stuart to be evaluated by a pediatric otolaryngologist, who felt a tonsillectomy was indicated.

Within three weeks of the tonsillectomy, Stuart's nocturnal enuresis was markedly reduced. By six weeks, it was gone altogether. While that in and of itself was a wonderfully positive outcome, what was most remarkable was his growth rebound. With the sleep apnea and its effect on sleep architecture and deep sleep eliminated, Stuart experienced a dramatic return to what was most likely his original growth trajectory. In the years following his surgery (the surgery was marked with the arrow on the chart on the next page), one can see his height begin to track back to the fiftieth percentile he had been in when the sleep disturbance presumably began.

---

* Since this is a book about kids, it's worth noting that Nightfall is a DC comic book character. Her powers are not what you think.

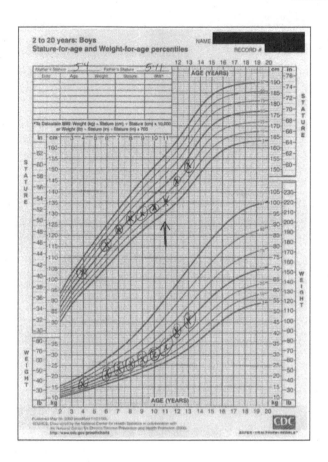

Don't Forget

1. Nocturnal enuresis is a common disorder in children.

2. Understand that while the disorder will generally get better over time, you do not have to passively wait before intervening.

3. Behavioral interventions are effective but labor-intensive interventions.

4. Sleep disorders in children can often precipitate episodes of nocturnal enuresis, so sleep evaluations should be a part of the evaluation for stubborn bed-wetting.

13

Snoring and Sleep Apnea

"He Has Grandma's Eyes and Grandpa's Compromised Breathing."

 Jack was an eleven-year-old who really liked baseball, in particular the Cleveland Indians. When he came to our office, every piece of clothing bore their logo. For a clinic that often features sleepy children, on the surface Jack was a far cry from sleepy.

He was accompanied by his mother, who was cheerful but obviously tired. After spending ten minutes with Jack, it was easy to see why. Jack was a very bright boy who had a lot to say about everything. While it is always fun to talk about baseball, it was very difficult to get Jack to focus on any questions about his sleep. At one point, I asked Jack how long it took him to fall asleep at night on average. About twenty minutes into his response, he broke down and began wailing about the Cleveland Indians logo and how on the one hand, he loved it and felt like it was a tribute to the native people of our land, but logically he knew it was offensive to many and needed to change. I decided to skip my questions about inattentiveness and emotional liability.

Jack's mother stated that over the last year, there had been dramatic changes in Jack. Emotionally, he was all over the place. Scholastically, he was typically a high achiever, but his motivation for school had waned. He was gaining weight and becoming self-conscious about it, which was not helped by new sporadic episodes of bed-wetting. "I am not sleeping over at anyone's house," he declared, anticipating that the topic might be brought up and wanting to nip it in the bud.

When asked about snoring, his mother said, "That's the reason we are here. His snoring has gotten so loud lately that we brought it up with his pediatric nurse practitioner and she immediately sent us to you.*

The snoring seemed to be developing in parallel with Jack's increasing weight. Jack was four foot seven inches but already weighed about 130 pounds, putting his BMI in the ninety-ninth percentile. Eating had become an issue, during the day and also at night, when he would wake up to eat. This had become so problematic that the cupboards and refrigerator had to be locked and healthy snacks for the night planned out.

The snoring was "scary," according to Jack's mother, with "terrible" sounds passing through bedroom walls with ease. "He frightens me. Sometimes I think he can't get oxygen to his brain." Snoring ran in the father's side of the family, so from Dad's perspective (he was not present), it was not a big deal and something Jack would eventually outgrow.

Jack's exam was totally unremarkable outside of his tonsils, which were the size of two autographed baseballs. They were red, mottled, and touching each other. I made a joke about them and wondered out loud how Jack was able to get any food in his stomach with two bowling balls blocking the way. Jack exclaimed, "I can feel them" as his mother told me that I was not the first person to remark about them. When I asked if he got frequent strep infections, Jack's mother said, "No. Everyone asks me that."

---

* Way to go, pediatric nurse practitioner!

We made Jack an appointment for a sleep study and a follow-up in our office to go over the results after it was complete.

~ ~ ~

Snoring. Outside of baldness, is there anything cuter in a baby and less attractive in an adult? Breathing disturbances make up a large portion of what pediatric sleep doctors deal with on a day-to-day basis. Despite the common nature of the problem, the pathway forward when dealing with a snoring child or teenager can often be quite murky.

What Are Snoring and Sleep Apnea?

Little baby snoring is adorable. As kids get older and some begin snoring loudly, the cuteness fades and suddenly you can have what sound likes a drunken professional wrestler sleeping in your eight-year-old's bedroom.*

Let's start things off with a seemingly easy question. What is snoring, and is it normal in a child? Snoring is the sound of vibrating airway tissue. As the breathing causes air to rush by structures in the airway, if those structures can move and oscillate, they can produce a sound, just like a plucked guitar string, though heinously more annoying. If we are defining "normal" in a strictly statistical manner, as in a normal distribution of children, it would be tough to call snoring abnormal, since some researchers would argue that most kids snore on occasion. My answer is yes, snoring all by itself (something we call primary snoring) is normal.

Sleep apnea, however, is not normal. Sleep apnea is what occurs when the vibrating airway starts to become the obstructed airway. In other words, instead of the airway just making noise, it begins to close off at night, preventing the child from getting oxygen. Brains love oxygen and do not fare well, even for short periods of time, if they are deprived of it. In fact, you could argue based upon the relative consumption of oxygen by the brain that our entire body is set up to basically provide a steady

* No disrespect to the men and women professional wrestlers out there. I'm not sure you snore any louder than the rest of us, but the image seemed like a good one.

source of oxygen to our greedy little brains. With sleep apnea, our brains face a difficult decision:

1. Sleep soundly and feel great the following day.

2. Breathe and not suffocate to death.

With sleep apnea, the brain has to decide which is more important. It can sleep or it can breathe, but it slowly loses the ability to do both effectively at the same time. Fortunately, your brain loves oxygen a bit more than sleep, so it chooses option #2, but in order to do that, it must constantly awaken throughout the night. Much like a dolphin skimming the surface of the water and periodically coming up for air as it swims, your child skims the surface of sleep, never going too deep because of the constant need to awaken to breathe.*

Sleep apnea is less common in children than it is in adults, but it is not rare, and the numbers have seemed to rise over the years. Currently it is thought that the condition affects 1 to 4 percent of children, with the most commonly affected age group being two- to eight-year-olds. This stems from the fact that proportionately, the tonsils of a five-year-old are quite large in relationship to their upper airway. As the child grows and her airway grows too, the tonsils do not tend to grow (and in some cases shrink), creating more space for breathing in the upper airway. For this reason, some adults display virtually no tonsillar tissue as they mature because of this shrinkage.

If you have at least one good ear, snoring should not be too difficult to detect in your child. In fact, his scoutmaster may have already hinted that he needs a "thicker tent." Detecting sleep apnea can be much more difficult if your child is not sleeping with you in bed or sharing the same

---

* Take a moment to think about the myriad problems that could arise if a child who is waking up frequently during the night to breathe is given a sedative to "help him sleep better at night." When a parent says, "The sleeping pill is working," what exactly is he saying? Could it be that by his definition of "work," the sleeping pill is merely allowing his child to suffocate longer?

room. Keep in mind that while snoring and sleep apnea often go hand in hand, there are often cases of quite profound pediatric sleep apnea that exist without significant or discernible snoring. In fact, a retrospective review of studies found that only looking at the clinical history (including snoring) in children was highly unreliable at detecting sleep apnea.

Symptoms of Snoring and Sleep Apnea

Anna Steese Richardson warned mothers about monitoring a child's breathing at night. "Irregular and unnatural breathing" should "give the inexperienced mother reason for quick action." She goes on to paint a fairly accurate picture of the symptoms of snoring and apnea in children and notes "breathing trouble; due to enlarged tonsils or adenoids, in which case the child is very restless, throwing itself from side to side, and often lying face downward." Even in the past, the picture of disturbed sleep from disturbed breathing was vivid.

Outside of listening to or recording your child's sleep (which can be very enlightening), how can parents make sure their child is not struggling with their breathing at night, particularly if snoring is not always a reliable marker for sleep apnea?

Let's start with the obvious, even though I know I just said it's not the only reliable indicator. The first thing to pay attention to is the nature of the snoring and breathing. Snoring is highly correlated with sleep apnea. In one Brazilian study, children who snored frequently and felt tired were three and a half times more likely to have sleep apnea.

We begin to worry about snoring crossing over from normal to abnormal when other criteria are met.

- Does your child do it sporadically, every now and then, or is she doing it every night? Keep in mind that only about one in ten children will snore every night, so if your child does, it is putting him in that 10 percent risk category for a more significant breathing disorder. In other words, that alone would not be considered normal.

- Does your child snore all night long or just for short periods of time? Is the snoring minimal or very loud? The timing and duration of snoring is something we look to for a measure of severity.

- Is there a positional component? Sometimes a child may snore only when on his back and not while on his side or propped up on a pillow.

- Does the snoring relate to allergies, colds, or other causes of congestion?

- Does your child seem to struggle with her breathing? Is the snoring erratic and punctuated by pauses or periods where she does not appear to be breathing?

These questions will help you probe the nature of your child's snoring and detect signs that it might be progressing from a simple inspiratory vibration to something more serious.

There are also symptoms that can emerge that are associated with snoring. These symptoms, often not directly linked to snoring, can be harbingers of bad things to come. As you think about your snoring child, does he exhibit the following symptoms:

- **Frequent nocturnal awakenings:** These awakenings can run the gamut from benign little arousals from which he immediately goes back to sleep to more disruptive awakenings in which your child is waking you up too.

- **Nightmares, night terrors, and other unusual behaviors at night:** These could be filed under the category of nocturnal awakenings, but sometimes they obscure the link between breathing and arousal at night. Often these behaviors disappear once the inciting event (the breathing disturbance) is identified and treated.

- **Enuresis/encopresis:** Bed-wetting and other accidents at night can be an indicator of breathing disturbances leading to arousal dysfunction at night.

- **Attention and hyperactivity issues:** Whether your child has been formally diagnosed with ADHD, is currently being evaluated, or there is simply a growing concern, disrupted sleep at night from breathing disturbances can play a big role contributing to or causing attention and concentration issues in your child. And where attention problems go . . .

- **Scholastic decline:** School problems follow. If your child is suddenly struggling in school, you may want to investigate your child's sleep and breathing a bit more aggressively. Boys, in particular those who develop excessive sleepiness from their breathing disturbances, are far more likely to be misdiagnosed with learning disorders. In fact, the combination of snoring, excessive sleepiness, and learning issues is a highly specific marker for sleep apnea.*

- **Diminished growth:** This is a tough one, but your pediatrician keeps a growth chart of your child. For me, it was the first assessment of my children about which I became competitive.† Because growth hormone is primarily secreted during deep sleep in children, if kids struggle to sleep and have diminished deep sleep, so too can their growth become diminished, leading to a

---

* In other words, when these three symptoms are present, you probably have a child with sleep apnea. Keep in mind, this symptom constellation is not very sensitive. In other words, if your child does not have those symptoms, it does not necessarily mean they do not have sleep apnea.

† Eighty-third percentile in height. That's a solid B.

child potentially falling off their current growth curve trajectory. I have seen many children address their breathing problems and almost immediately experience a growth surge.

Keep in mind, these symptoms are often associated with a child who snores, but the absence of snoring does not rule out the diagnosis of sleep apnea. If these aforementioned symptoms are present in your child, consider a sleep evaluation even if your child sleeps quietly.

Diagnosing Sleep Apnea

The diagnosis of sleep apnea requires a sleep study. Currently, there are two different types of sleep studies: the in-lab sleep study (or in-lab polysomnogram) and the home sleep test. While the home sleep test is mainly aimed at diagnosing sleep apnea, it is generally not approved by insurance plans for use on children. Because of a child's higher tendency to knock or pull sensors off during the night, in-lab studies attended by a technician who can make sure the study goes smoothly are preferred. More information about the ins and outs of a sleep study can be found in chapter 17.

During the sleep study, your child will be monitored for many things, breathing among them. Sleep apnea is fundamentally a disruption of your child's ability to breathe. The sleep disturbance is the natural outcome of those breathing interruptions, so assessing and quantifying the breathing disturbances is important.

During the sleep study, your child will have several devices attached to her.

A nasal cannula (or tube) will be placed underneath her nose/mouth to measure how much air she is exhaling. In some labs, the change in air pressure is utilized to make this measurement. It is usually labeled as nasal pressure transducer airflow (PTAF) in a sleep study. In other labs, a device that measures temperature change called a thermistor is used. It works because exhaled air is warmed by the body, so the change in temperature between the warm exhaled air and cooler inhaled air creates the wave. The wave it creates typically has a smoother appearance.

When the child breathes in, the tracing goes up (referred to as a negative deflection), and during exhalation, the tracing goes down (a positive deflection). In the following example, you can see the child has taken eight breaths in thirty seconds.

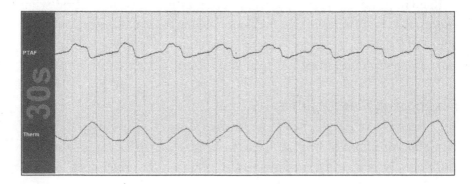

During a sleep study, we look for changes in breathing patterns. In the case of sleep apnea, we are looking for places where your child's breathing is diminished or absent altogether. While that is a difficult thing to see sometimes when you are looking at thirty seconds of data as per the previous graph . . .

It is quite easy to see when you zoom out and look at five minutes of breathing.

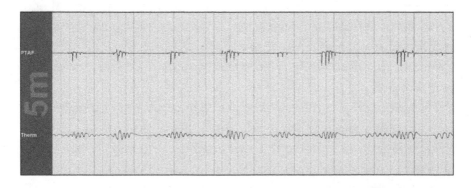

The thermistor and PTAF are indicators of the air your child is moving in and out of their nose/mouth. If we follow the path of that air, we know that the oxygen that is breathed in eventually gets to the lungs, which allow the oxygen to diffuse into the blood. Fortunately, we can measure how much oxygen is dissolved in the bloodstream of your child.

The pulse oximeter is a simple device that is clipped onto the finger, and it measures how much oxygen is being carried by the blood. Most people have had the little red light attached to their finger at some point or another. Generally speaking, a normal value is 97 to 99 percent. During a sleep study, a child's pulse oximeter value is measured constantly all night long. Ideally, it looks like this:

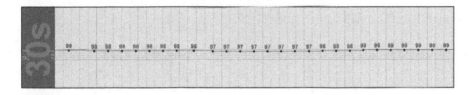

Now, let's look at what happens when we add a pulse oximeter to the PTAF and thermistor tracing in a child with breathing problems.

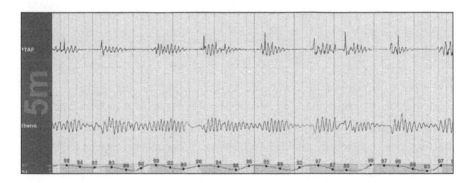

Again, you can easily see the breathing interruptions, but now, a few beats after the breathing disturbance, there is a drop in oxygen. And as we have talked about many times, since your brain loves oxygen, there is a rapid upswing back to normal once the child awakens and resumes normal breathing. Counting about eight breathing disruptions in five minutes of this child's sleep, you can imagine the volume of sleep disruptions were this pattern to continue all night!

Two more pieces of equipment that you might notice during a sleep study are the elastic bands around your child's chest and abdomen.

Before we talk about the function of these bands, take a moment to think about your own breathing. Look down at your chest and belly and take a deep breath in. Notice how your chest puffs out? Now breathe out. Look at how your body seems to deflate and become smaller. These bands, when they stretch and contract, can take that physical change and turn it into a waveform we can measure, just like the breathing devices we mentioned earlier. By doing this, these bands can measure the effort your child is making when she breathes.

Typically, when breathing is normal, they seem to mirror the wave patterns of the thermistor and PTAF.

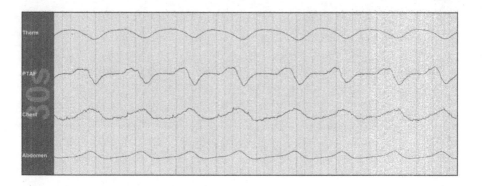

However, when breathing becomes problematic, the output from the bands can be very helpful in determining the nature of the breathing disturbance your child may be exhibiting, since sleep apnea can be obstructive or central. In obstructive sleep apnea, the child is attempting to breathe, but there is an obstruction preventing that from happening. During the study, you see the amount of air the child is moving from their mouth (PTAF, Therm) flatline, but the chest and abdomen are still showing signs that the child is working hard to breathe as their chest and abdomen move in and out.

For children, we consider a breathing disturbance significant if there is a reduction of flow (in thermistor or PTAF) by 90 percent or more, for two breaths or more, despite ongoing respiratory effort. Look at the example above. It appears that the PTAF and thermistor signals completely disappear and flatline (that's more than 90 percent). You can also see that

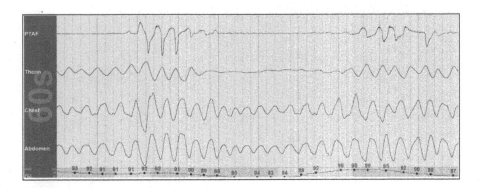

it looks like the breathing is absent for eight to nine breaths—far more than two. Finally, you can see the breathing effort in the chest and abdominal leads is maintained.

In central sleep apnea, the airway is clear of any obstruction, yet the body is not breathing.

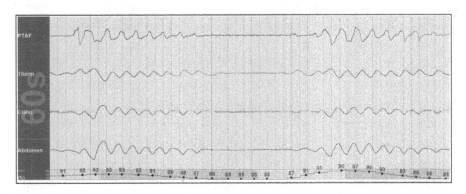

What you have seen at this point is how we as sleep specialists can measure and count the number of breathing disturbances your child has at night.

Treatment of Snoring and Sleep Apnea

Theoretically, the treatment of snoring and sleep apnea is easy—for snoring, just stop the vibration, for sleep apnea, just keep the airway from collapsing. Simple, right? Not exactly, especially in a kid. What kid wants to bring a breathing device to a sleepover party?

There is a level of nuance when it comes to the treatment of sleep apnea in children, especially when the diagnostic criteria is essentially anyone having more than one breathing problem/hour. Because of the criteria, an incredibly wide diagnostic spectrum is created.

When a child has sleep apnea, they could have 1.4 breathing disturbances per hour, or they could theoretically have 180 per hour (each breathing disturbance must last ten seconds with a ten-second gap in between). That is a huge range. It is the difference between having one to two migraines every year to having one every day.

As a physician and someone whose job it is to guide a family through the entire process of their sleep evaluation, this can be tricky. I find that in many cases, the diagnosis of any sleep apnea is the nail and the medical response is the hammer. What I mean by that is the sleep apnea diagnosis needs to be properly put into context to get the proper response.

To do that, several things need to happen. The first is that your child needs to have an in-lab attended sleep study. After that study, and this is important, there should be an appointment where you and the sleep specialist sit down and talk about the sleep study. In some situations, a pediatrician, primary care doctor, ENT, or other non–sleep specialist will order the study. When this happens, some other sleep doctor will read the study and report: *sleep apnea*, or *no sleep apnea*. As stated, sleep apnea can mean a lot of things, and the individual sleep situation your child is in deserves specific attention. Unfortunately, when this happens, the non–sleep specialist who ordered the study may not appreciate the nuances associated with sleep apnea. What was the motivating factor behind the sleep study? Snoring in an otherwise healthy child? Witnessed breathing disturbances? A child with frequent night terrors, bed-wetting, and near constant strep infections? These pretest characteristics coupled with the relative severity of the sleep apnea, the changes in oxygen during the night, as well as the age and stage of development of the child create a complicated decision-making matrix that should be discussed with an expert.

As far as treatments for sleep apnea in children go, the options are few. Surgery, typically a tonsillectomy, is the most common route for treatment. For children with significant overbites, dental manipulation via braces or surgery can be effective. Incidentally, I have seen cases where children were most likely given sleep apnea after their underbites were corrected. Finally, as with the majority of adults, continuous positive airway pressure (CPAP) devices can be used. I think for the average child, this is a tall order. That said, I am often surprised by how capable they are in terms of using these devices when necessary.

One of the benefits of a CPAP device is that it's temporary. This is important because with some young children, as time passes, they can outgrow the disorder. As their stature increases and the relative size and proportion of the upper airway changes, the dynamics of their breathing can shift enough to improve the sleep apnea. Newer CPAP devices can help specialists track the severity of a child's breathing disturbance. In some cases, a child's breathing can improve to the point of no longer needing the CPAP. A follow-up sleep study can be done in cases like this, or post-surgery, to ensure resolution of the disorder.

In some kids, particularly those who have mild cases in which symptoms are minimal, treatment may not be necessary. With these children, symptoms should be monitored via routine follow-up with a sleep specialist. In some cases, weight loss and adjusting the sleeping position of the child (tilting his head up) can be helpful.

 Jack could not have been more excited about the sleep study. The only hitch with the night in the lab was that he insisted on bringing heavier flannel-type Cleveland Indians pajamas in the middle of the summer, so sweating was a problem. Outside of this small struggle, Jack did a fantastic job during the night, and his sleep study was quite surprising.

This is five minutes of Jack's sleep. Now that you know about how breathing is measured on a sleep study, take a look at the Therm and PTAF tracings during this study. Notice the breathing followed by the flatline pauses—Jack had a lot of them. Furthermore, during these episodes, his oxygen dropped considerably. Seeing breathing like this in young kids in never easy.

Jack ended up having almost forty such breathing disturbances per hour. Forget the pediatric criteria for sleep apnea. Jack would be considered severe on the adult scale.

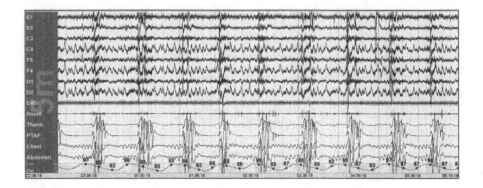

The bright side is that we figured it out. We have a fixable problem here. After discussing the available options, they decided to get input from a local ENT who has a reputation for being very conservative when it comes to tonsillectomies (which I think is great). I frequently send him kids I think have big tonsils and his notes back to me are the medical equivalent of "meh." Not this time. He was impressed enough to recommend immediate surgery.

And that is what Jack got—a tonsillectomy and lots of ice cream. As with many kids who have significant sleep apnea, the changes that happened in Jack after treatment were impressive. Jack's sleep improved within a week or two after surgery. His weight had dropped by four pounds at our first follow-up visit, and his behavior and achievement in school were improved. The bed-wetting stopped immediately and never returned. Later that year, the Cleveland Indians went to the World Series. It was a good year for Jack.

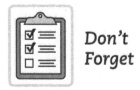

Don't Forget

1. Despite its positioning in chapter 13, sleep apnea is a common and important sleep problem in children.

2. Sleep apnea and snoring are not necessarily tied together. A child can snore but not have sleep apnea, have sleep apnea but not snore, or have both.

3. If you have a sleep study, sit down and talk to the doctor who read the study. Every sleep apnea diagnosis does not require surgery or a CPAP!

4. In some more unusual cases, sleep apnea is happening not because your child can't breathe but rather because his brain won't breathe. Central sleep apnea should be dealt with by a sleep specialist.

Sleep and Special Situations

You Are Now Entering a World of Total Medical Confusion and Misinformation. Please Buckle Up.

The first time I saw Charity, she was looking at our office copy of the newest *Vanity Fair* magazine. Despite being nonverbal, she went through every page, and if there was a woman in a dress pictured, she would point and make a kind of, *Ooooh, I like that* sound and smile. Each time she looked to her mother for approval, and each time her mother gave a short but impressively thoughtful answer. "Yes, that is a nice dress." "Oh, that is flattering." "I'm not sure you could call that a dress." "Oh God, that's dreadful."

Charity is a sixteen-year-old with Down syndrome and significant developmental delay and cognitive/language impairments. She was referred to my clinic because of headaches diagnosed by a very astute developmental pediatrician. The headaches were initially thought to be migraines, but their lack of response to typical migraine medications were concerning. Charity has a small airway and snores loudly during the night, and her sleep disturbances led to the referral.

In addition to the snoring and sleep apnea, Charity does not sleep much. She is always the last to go to sleep in the family and the first to awaken in the morning. Charity's mom had gotten used to the schedule but always feels slightly uncomfortable about whether her daughter is getting adequate rest.

After our meeting and with an agreement that Charity could keep the *Vanity Fair*, we arranged for her to have an overnight sleep study.

~ ~ ~

There are a variety of medical situations that can create unique sleep issues for children. These issues can be temporary, or they can present lifelong challenges for you and your child, particularly when applying standards and practices meant for average children to your exceptional one. This chapter will look at the unique sleep challenges these kids have, what current research says about sleep in these conditions, and practical advice for helping them achieve the sleep they need.

Down Syndrome

Approximately 50 percent of children with Down syndrome have sleep problems. These children can have behavioral issues surrounding sleep (insomnia, anxiety) as well as physical obstacles (sleep apnea) that can create a confusing picture of sleepiness and inability to sleep.

Because of the high prevalence of breathing disturbances in this population, I feel all patients with Down syndrome should be evaluated with an in-lab sleep study. Early sleep intervention can improve both the long-term health and intellectual achievement of these individuals.

Autism Spectrum Disorder

Sleep disturbances have been reported in as many as 80 percent of children with autism spectrum disorder, with 35 to 40 percent reporting difficulty falling asleep or maintaining sleep. This is a trait shared among children with many neurogenetic disorders. In fact, atypical insomnia may be a presenting sign of autism in young children. Unusually frequent awakenings can precede the diagnosis of autism by as much as one year. While numerous studies indicate that children with autism awaken more frequently during the night, studies show that they may only be awakening one to two more times per night than children without autism, so detection can be difficult. These disruptions are not without consequence though, as the sleep disorders in these children are often associated with higher incidence of inattention, irritability, hyperactive behaviors, and even physical aggression.

New evidence is emerging that restless legs syndrome may contribute to the problem, with RLS occurring in as many as 39 percent of cases of children with autism who are also struggling with insomnia.

Advocating for sleep disorder screening, even in those with milder forms of autism spectrum disorder, may help significantly improve problem daytime behaviors.

Rhythmic movement disorder, discussed in chapter 10, is often seen in the autism population and can result in injury, particularly when the movement is head banging.

Traumatic Head Injuries and Concussions

Children who have suffered injuries to the head or concussions are susceptible to sleep disturbances and signs of excessive sleepiness both immediately after the incident, and for prolonged periods of time after the event, even in cases where the child otherwise seems to have recovered completely. A recent study indicated that younger children may be more vulnerable to these changes than older children.

Epilepsy

Sleep disorders are one of the most prevalent symptomatic complaints in epilepsy, and unfortunately one of the most neglected, even by medical professionals. Nocturnal seizures can often be the heralding sign of an underlying seizure disorder, yet they are often exceptionally difficult to recognize, secondary to their vastly different ways of presenting.

There are several seizure disorders that typically begin in childhood and feature nocturnal symptoms/seizures. One of the most common seizure disorders is benign epilepsy of childhood with central-temporal spikes (formerly benign rolandic epilepsy). During the day, these children often exhibit twitching, numbness, or facial tingling that can cause drooling and speech impairment. Further confusing the picture is its very distinct brain wave pattern at night. These kids tend to have a preponderance of their seizures—70 to 80 percent—during sleep. These seizures, and the observed sleep disturbances, often lead to improper diagnosis.

Juvenile myoclonic epilepsy (JME) is another sleep-related epilepsy seen in adolescence. Its telltale symptom is jerks or seizures, usually within one to two hours upon awakening from sleep or even a nap. These events can sometimes mistakenly be attributed to a sleep disorder when they happen close to awakening. Moreover, sleep deprivation is a known risk factor for children with JME having seizures. Ensuring adequate and high-quality sleep is of paramount importance to these children.

While seizures are relatively rare causes of sleep disturbances, consider the diagnosis in any child with frequent and repetitive awakenings during the night.

Bipolar Mood Disorder

Several studies indicate that children with bipolar mood disorder are far more susceptible to sleep disorders including insomnia, bedtime resistance, parasomnias, and circadian rhythm disorders. In a recent study made up of twenty-one bipolar patients under the age of twenty-four, 41 percent reported poor sleep quality. A focused sleep assessment, behavioral sleep evaluation, and circadian intervention should be considered in all such children. Polysomnographic evaluation (a sleep study) is generally indicated for children struggling with sleep.

A consistent finding among bipolar patients is that it takes them longer to fall asleep. Once asleep, patients with bipolar mood disorder tend to sleep less at night and possibly more during the day, according to a 2020 study. The greatest reduction of sleep happens between 12:00 a.m. and 6:00 a.m. Other studies have suggested that their denser REM periods are electrographical evidence of this reduced sleep need.

In my experience, these sleep interventions are often ignored, as mental-health professionals choose sedation instead, the rationale being "healthy sleep is essential for optimal treatment of their psychiatric disorder." While I do not disagree with this motivation at all, I do have an issue with the assumption that the use of trazodone, Seroquel, clonaz-epam, or other sedating psychoactive medications constitutes an intervention leading to "healthy sleep." In other words, sedation and sleep are not the same thing.

The presence of mania is a confounding situation. When a bipolar patient is acutely manic, they temporarily break the "everybody sleeps" rule, and potentially may need to be sedated as this is often a dangerous situation for a child to be in. While sedation may be warranted in certain acute situations, in general, it is an inappropriate treatment policy for nightly sleep outside of a crisis. Parents should be vigilant and not be afraid to question nonemergent nightly sedation without a sleep specialist consultation or ongoing involvement.

Vitamin and Nutritional Deficiencies

Disorders in this category are going to be rare finds. The likelihood that a child would have such significant dietary deficiencies as to create sleep problems is probably going to have more obvious and significant problems than sleep difficulties.

Despite this, it is worth considering the following:

Iron: Low iron can lead to anemia, and it can cause a sense of lethargy and fatigue. Low iron is also a contributor to restless legs syndrome.

Fatty acids: There is some evidence that children deficient in long-chain omega-3 fatty acids such as docosahexaenoic acid can sleep better when they receive omega-3 supplementation. One study of seven- to nine-year-old children showed omega-3 supplementation led to fifty-eight more minutes of sleep on average, and fewer awakenings.

Magnesium: Magnesium is known to increase the GABA levels in the brain, a calming neurotransmitter. Despite weak evidence in adults, there is no compelling evidence that it improves the sleep of children despite reports that magnesium is often underconsumed in children.

Charity was a superstar patient during the sleep study. My technician sent me a text the next day saying what an amazing patient she turned out to be. In the video of the sleep study, Charity was clearly reading the *Vanity Fair* from my office as the electrodes were attached to her scalp.

Her sleep study ended up showing significant sleep apnea that was remedied by a tonsillectomy and an attempted ultrasound reduction of her tongue size, both done in an effort to create more airway space. The surgery brought her apnea index down from approximately thirty breathing disturbances per hour to eleven.

The sleep study additionally showed episodes of bradycardia that were, until that point, undiscovered. This slower heart rhythm led to episodes of heart block that were picked up by the technician as well. She was referred to a cardiologist, who was able to address her cardiac issues.

After the sleep apnea surgery, Charity had significantly fewer headaches, which allowed her mother to take her off two of her medications. According to her mother, Charity became less frustrated and emotional after the intervention.

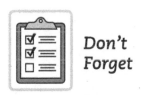

Don't Forget

1. Sleep problems play a major role in many conditions.

2. Often, a sleep evaluation can lead to interventions that improve the severity and treatment response of the parent disorder.

15

Disorders of Fatigue

Why Your Kid Is Exhausted (and Not Depressed)

Keisha is a sixteen-year-old girl who came to my clinic with her mother. She has been struggling with feeling tired for one to two years, and the symptoms are slowly getting worse. Once a promising young gymnast, she simply does not have the motivation or ability to participate in the sport, stating that it has gotten so bad, "I can barely pull myself up onto the uneven bars." Doctors and coaches have diagnosed her with anxiety and chronic fatigue disorder, and she does have a remote history of an eating disorder. Mom added a long history of issues that are related to the fact that "Keisha needs more sleep." She had read an article about Olympic gymnasts needing more sleep and stated that she knew if Keisha could get more sleep, "This would all be taken care of." Her medication list features two medications I call SSPs (secret sleeping pills), named so because they carry no formal FDA approval for sleep but are often used in particular doses at night to sedate). In her case she was on trazodone (an FDA-approved antidepressant) and a small dose of Seroquel (an FDA-approved mood stabilizer and antipsychotic). Nothing was helping, and if anything, it was "making things worse."

"When you say nothing helped, what exactly do you mean?" I asked. For caregivers who have children with difficult issues, it is important to define therapy goals. Help what? Help her win a gold medal on the vault? Simply make it to practice? Feel somewhat more normal?

"None of it helps her sleep."

~ ~ ~

In my humble opinion, there is no more important topic within the world of sleep than the symptom of fatigue. I'm sure you are asking yourself the question, "If it is so important, how did it end up near the end of the book?" Totally fair question, and the answer is simple: to fully understand fatigue in a child, you first must be an expert in sleep.*

The Difference Between Sleepy and Fatigued

Before we jump into fatigue, I want to briefly touch on a word: "tired." "Tired" is an important word because your child is 99.99 percent more likely to use the word "tired" to describe how he feels than "fatigued."

Likely: "Mommy, I feel tired and my tummy hurts bad."

Unlikely: "Mother, I am sensing some epigastric discomfort accompanied by substantial fatigue of an unknown etiology."

When I think of the word "tired," I think of an umbrella:

* Which you undoubtedly are by now.

"Tired" is a general word many kids use to express a range of feelings. In my life, the main two symptoms that fall under this vague term are sleepiness and fatigue.

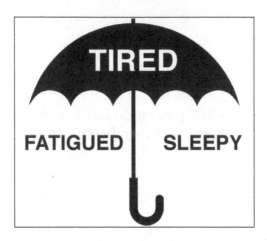

A quick note: I've used the word "tired" because it is the word your kids will use the most. "I'm tired and I want to go to bed." You can substitute all kinds of words for tired: "pooped," "worn-out," "beat," "fried," "blasted," "annihilated," "spent," "done," etc. They are all similarly poorly defined words.

So why does it matter if a tired child is sleepy or if she is fatigued? It matters a lot. Up until this point, we have spent a significant amount of time talking about sleep and disorders of sleep. Much of this book is made up of diagnoses that take wonderful restorative sleep and ruin it. The result is a sleepy child—a child who is seeking (and in many cases, acquiring) sleep at times when they should not be. In other words, what is going on when a kid falls asleep during chemistry class? Their brain is so in need of sleep, for some reason or another, that they are doing it inches from a Bunsen burner.

Sleepiness is an excessive drive to sleep. It happens because a person is either (1) lacking sufficient sleep quantity (chapter 5), or (2) lacking sufficient sleep quality (pretty much the rest of this book). It does not have to be pathological. The sleepiness we feel at the end of a busy day is perfectly appropriate. Excessive sleepiness during the day, by definition, is typically pathological . . . it indicates a problem. A problem I attempt to fix every day. A problem I hope this book is helping you solve with your child.

Let's turn our attention to fatigue. Fatigue is important because it is often talked about in the same ways as sleepiness. The words are used interchangeably, and because of this, a disorder of fatigue can quickly and easily get pushed down the disorder of sleepiness pathway.

What is fatigue? In a word: energy. Fatigue is why you stop after nine bench press reps, when your goal had been eleven. Your muscles simply do not have it in them to push that weight anymore at this moment. Usually, a period of rest will restore your muscles' energy and you can continue. On a cellular level, it has everything to do with energy available to the mitochondria. It is gasoline in a fuel tank. When it is empty, the system slows dramatically or stops. Notice how I never mentioned sleep, or drive to sleep. You didn't fail to lift the weight on those last two bench press reps because you were nodding off on the bench . . . or simply overcome by sleepiness. No. You are wide awake, screaming things like, "I got this, baby" to your spotter who is in turn yelling back to you, "This is all you, baby." Nobody is exactly yawning in this situation.

When I work with patients who have complicated issues, I step back, take stock of this overall situation, and try to encapsulate it all into "the bullet." The bullet is ideally one sentence that fully introduces and describes a patient's problem, and formulating it is an art. You learn quickly in medical school and beyond, some have it and some do not.* Here's my bullet:

- Keisha is a sixteen-year-old with a persistent and relatively chronic issue of fatigue over the last two to three years.

* When my kids were small and they would read a book, I would often ask them for the bullet. Answers varied dramatically, with Harry Potter books being incredibly difficult for kids to summarize in a sentence. I do remember my daughter tackling Tolkien, and when she was done, I asked her for the bullet. Undaunted, she replied, "Basically a Harry Potter rip-off."

Looking at this bullet, who said anything about sleep? Exploring her sleep history, she has had issues with sleep onset, but the medications have helped with that significantly. Probing further, the next logical question becomes, "What time do you go to bed, Keisha?"

"Nine p.m."

Remember that sixteen-year-old who liked to get to bed around 9:00 p.m.? Yeah, neither do I. Any time I have a teenager going to bed before the major networks are allowed to air crime dramas, that's a red flag.

"Before you started taking the meds you are on, how long would it take you to fall asleep?"

"Usually an hour, sometimes longer."

"Why not go to bed then . . . when it seems like your body naturally wants to sleep?"

Confused looks from both mother and daughter.

"Because I'm so tired."

Houston, we have a problem.

All too often, there is a relationship that is forged in the minds of patients who struggle with fatigue. They wake up in the morning, stretch, and immediately experience that all-too-familiar feeling of fatigue as soon as they wake up. At that point, they look backward over their shoulder and think, *Ugh, if I could have just slept better/more, I wouldn't feel this way.*

Maybe . . . but maybe not.

Put a different way, over time there becomes a great and focused effort to treat an individual's fatigue by improving their sleep. This is kind of like treating someone's heartache over the loss of a loved one with the nitro we give heart attack patients for chest pain. Not exactly the same kind of heartache.

Do I have an issue with improving Keisha's sleep? Absolutely not. Even if that does not solve the problems she is having, I'm all for making someone's sleep better. Two minor problems:

1. Is giving a sixteen-year-old trazodone and Seroquel really improving her sleep, or are we simply sedating her?

2. Are we certain Keisha has sleep that needs improving? What evidence exists that there is a sleep problem we need to fix?

Having read this book, you already know the answer to #1. If you would like me to summarize the body of research studies that convincingly shows how either of these drugs are improving Keisha's sleep, unfortunately I can't. No such studies exist. She has been given these drugs not only because Keisha and her mother don't understand the difference between sleepiness and fatigue, but also because the doctors treating her do not either. And believe me, a sixteen-year-old with a motivated mother and an iPhone can see a ton of specialists in two years. Phrases like, "She has to get her sleep in order to get better," and "Her fatigue represents poor sleep, so we need to remedy that to allow her body to heal" and equally vacuous phrases fill their heads, so of course we can't have Keisha taking an hour to fall asleep every night! No wonder she's so tired.

See the problem? There has been a determination here that is highly erroneous, and the logic flows like this:

Keisha is tired and fatigued. TRUE
It takes a while for Keisha to fall asleep. TRUE
If we can get Keisha to sleep faster, she will no longer feel fatigued
    and tired. FALSE

From everything you have read thus far, you know that in general, people with a sleep disorder want more sleep, not less sleep. You also know that people need different amounts of sleep. An alternate way of looking at this situation is:

Keisha is tired and fatigued. TRUE
It takes a while for Keisha to fall asleep because she is going to bed
    before she has become sufficiently sleepy to fall asleep. TRUE
Keisha's sleep is actually pretty normal and that's why she does not
    feel particularly sleepy, just fatigued. TRUE

We should move on from the sleep evaluation and focus in on
   causes of fatigue in Keisha. TRUE

Keisha really does not have a primary sleep disorder. She never did, at
least when this process began. She may have one now that we have accidentally convinced her that she needs to be asleep by 9:00 p.m. to be
healthy, and that she needs drugs for her sleep to be restorative. It is a
terrible thing to go to bed every night with your health on the line.

In Keisha's case, I felt like it was important to do a sleep study on her
to give a more objective assessment of her sleep quality. For difficult and
protracted illnesses like Keisha's, I like to be as confident as possible
when I report back to the family and the referring physician. My hunches
have been wrong before, so it is nice to have something concrete to back
things up.

At this point, my job changes. I go from the guy who is going to solve
the medical mystery and tell you what the diagnosis is to the guy who
can't tell you what it is, but he can help you cross off what it isn't from the
list. Not as good as being the hero, but at least we are making progress.

Armed with the normal sleep study, normal Epworth Sleepiness Scale,
and the absolute lack of meaningful change in her sleep once the sleep
aids were scrapped and she was allowed to go to bed when her body was
actually sleepy, the question remains . . . why is Keisha fatigued?

Compared to fatigue, sleepiness is a breeze. If someone is sleepy, as
I've said before, they are dealing with an inadequate amount or a diminished quality of sleep. Neither of these are terribly difficult to determine.
With fatigue, it is a whole other story. One time, when I was giving a
lecture, I proclaimed that you could write a book several inches thick
filled with the nearly endless causes of a kid's fatigue. I even went so far
as to claim that there were causes for every letter of the alphabet, at
which point an audience member yelled out, "Name them." I tried on
the spot and was crushing it, until I got to J and was stumped.

That night, still stewing about my missed opportunity to wow the
audience and make an important point at the same time, I created the list
in about twenty minutes with many letters having multiple alternates:
Here they are . . .

Anemia
B_{12} deficiency
Cancer
Congestive heart failure
COPD
COVID-19
Cushing's disease
Depression
Diabetes
Electrolyte disorder
Fibromyalgia
Grief
Hormone deficiency
Iron deficiency
Joubert syndrome
Kidney disease
Lyme disease
Mononucleosis
Multiple sclerosis
Nephrotic syndrome
Organophosphate poisoning
POTS
Pregnancy
Q fever
Rheumatoid arthritis
Scurvy
Scarlet fever
Strep throat
Thyroid disorder
Uremia
Varicella (chicken pox)
Whooping cough
Xanthine oxidase deficiency
Yersiniosis
Zika virus

The point of the list and this chapter is this: There are lots of causes of fatigue. Loads and loads of potential diagnoses. If the doctor treating your child's fatigue is out of options, it is time to find another doctor. "We've checked everything" is never true because the list of everything is virtually endless. What they are really saying is "We have checked everything we know about." It is like asking me why your car won't start.

"Do you have the key?"

"Yes."

"Does your car have gas in it?"

"Yes"

"Is the car in park?"

"Yes."

"Is the battery on your car charged and attached?"

"Yes."

"Is the alternator okay?"

"Yes."

At this point, I'm out of ideas. I have ruled out a few easy things, but it is time to take your car to a specialist, because you have reached the edge of my knowledge. Just because I don't know the answer does not mean the answer does not exist.

And so it goes with fatigue. At this point, we ended up referring Keisha to another specialist who dealt exclusively with fatigue in children. She was eventually diagnosed both with a more unusual tick-borne illness and potentially some food intolerances. A course of antibiotics along with a diet that eliminated wheat seemed to cure Keisha in a relatively rapid period of time.

It was always bothersome to me that she had two unusual diagnoses: tick and wheat sensitivity. The neurologist nerd in me wanted to know the real answer: Tick? Bread? Chance?

This story is fun because Keisha came back to my clinic years later, still doing quite well. She felt strongly that it was wheat all along and that the tick illness was irrelevant.

"Every now and then I convince myself that it was all in my head, and I stuff myself with pizza and bread, and every time, I pay the price," she said. "It was the wheat. I have no idea why it started when it did, but I hate it."

I thought it appropriate to include a chapter on fatigue in children because I want you educated, armed, and ready when you see your primary care provider. I want you to understand that while a thyroid panel, B$_{12}$, blood glucose, and test for mononucleosis are a great place to start, these tests coming back normal by no means indicate that you are finished in this workup for fatigue, and there is lots of work to be done.

Chronic Fatigue Syndrome

One final thought about fatigue. Within this world is the diagnosis of chronic fatigue syndrome (CFS). I want to talk about this diagnosis and, in particular, its designation as a "syndrome" and not a typical disease.

There are a lot of syndromes in medicine, and they usually carry with them a strange, hard-to-define stigma. Irritable bowel syndrome, polycystic ovary syndrome, postural orthostatic tachycardia syndrome (POTS), complex regional pain syndrome, and fibromyalgia syndrome (the syndrome is often dropped). In children, there are a wealth of syndromes, often referring to genetic abnormalities (Down syndrome, Klinefelter's syndrome, Rett syndrome).

What is a syndrome, and how does it differ from a disease? In general, a disease is a medical disorder with a known underlying cause or pathophysiology, and potentially a definitive treatment. We know the root of the problem basically, even if it cannot be fixed or treated.

Take diabetes, for instance. Diabetes is the shortened form of the disease's full name, diabetes mellitus. This is derived from the Greek *diabetes* "to siphon" and Latin *mellitus,* meaning "sweetened." Literally a sweet liquid siphoned from the body because in diabetes, sugar is dumped into the urine rather than being appropriately taken in by the cells of your body. We worked out the underlying cause of the disorder, the role of the pancreas and insulin, in the late 1800s/early 1900s. Treatments were soon to follow. Boom: a disease complete with a scientifically validated mechanism that explains all the symptoms (characteristic changes in blood sugar, retinopathy, fruity breath, kidney damage, coma) and hints at a cure (figure out a way to help the body make insulin or be less resistant to insulin).

Unfortunately, syndromes are not so straightforward. An individual with chronic fatigue syndrome (CFS) is tired all the time for no clear reason. The thyroid test, blood sugar test, mono test, Lyme disease test, and sleep test have all come back normal. Like a coffee shop punch card, once you've collected your nine normal tests, the diagnosis of chronic fatigue syndrome is free!

The problem with myalgic encephalomyelitis (another name for the disorder, so named perhaps to help legitimize the condition in the eyes of those who don't recognize it as being a real entity) is that it does not have a typical disease process like diabetes. More important, it lacks any discernible cure or effective treatment. It is a condition that affects millions of people of all ages, costs our economy an estimated seventeen to twenty-four billion dollars each year in health-related expenses and lost earned income, and it has virtually nonexistent diagnostic criteria. Doctors often refer to this condition as a "wastebasket" diagnosis. In other words, it catches all the trash not being filed in other diagnostic folders.

Doctors can be a strange bunch when it comes to things they do not understand. For many, instead of seeing it as a puzzle or an opportunity, they see it as a frustration . . . perhaps even a bizarre questioning of their diagnostic abilities. For this reason, some doctors can be quite cruel when there are disorders happening outside of what they are capable of explaining. They can be dismissive and accusatory. Your child is faking. You are not parenting properly. The list goes on.

I have absolutely no problem telling you right now that not only are there many things in medicine I don't know or cannot explain, but there are also many things in sleep that I cannot explain. Sometimes people have a way of simply not fitting neatly into a diagnostic category. And so it is with chronic fatigue syndrome.

Is CFS real? I think it is, but in many ways (and based upon its diagnostic criteria) it is a diagnosis of exclusion. What this means is to make the diagnosis, you need to have good guidance for ruling out all of the other "diseases" and various causes of chronic fatigue before you can make the CFS call and feel good about it.

And if you do it the right way, you should feel good about it. Just because someone can't necessarily cure your child's CFS does not mean it is not real, just as my inability to explain the popularity of taking pictures of the food you order at restaurants does not make it any less popular. Once the diagnosis is made, this often helps to provide a road map for moving forward with interventions to minimize the syndrome's impact.

One parting note. I have no idea why your child developed chronic fatigue syndrome. CFS is unfair. Breaking your leg in a football game making a big tackle really sucks, but cruising into school on crutches, getting tons of attention and sympathy, having the guy you like sign your cast . . . all pretty awesome. Slinking into class late because you felt too exhausted to get out of bed and having to stumble through an explanation of CFS . . . not exactly the same thing. It is not fair. I will say this—not that I'm approaching "old doctor" status—but through the years I have seen the disorder disappear as strangely and inexplicably as it appeared. In fact, I see it all the time. I'll run into a parent in a grocery store, and if they recognize me, they will often tell me how their kid, my former patient, is heading off to the Naval Academy on a rowing scholarship and how a few years after our meeting, the condition just seemed to get better. There is hope. Find a pediatrician who has an aggressive approach to fatigue or see a fatigue specialist. Do everything they tell you to do to help get your child's symptoms under control, and don't give up hope!

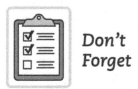

Don't Forget

1. Doctors often see disorders of fatigue as being the same as disorders of sleepiness. They are not.

2. When disorders of fatigue are misdiagnosed and mistreated as sleep disorders, issues generally get worse.

16

Time to See a Sleep Specialist

Pediatric Sleep Doctor—It's Totally a Real Thing!

At some point, you may determine that simply reading this book or watching some YouTube videos about your kid's sleep are not enough to solve your child's underlying sleep disorder. It's okay. There are not only many things that we did not cover in this book, but there are also reasons for collecting more sleep data on your child than you could easily do at home.

Merely knowing that there are sleep disorder specialists who can treat your child's sleep problem properly is a huge leap forward. For many people, the idea of their child seeing a sleep specialist or having a sleep study is not something that they are aware of as an option.

Unfortunately, at the time of this book's writing, the term "sleep specialist" can mean many things, from a doctor who has spent many years studying neurology and the science of sleep, to a person who has acquired an online designation as "sleep coach." The landscape is wide open and terribly unregulated.

Part of my motivation for writing this book is that the number of well-qualified physicians who treat the full range of kid-specific sleep disorders is small, and unfortunately those numbers are being dwarfed by the growing number of "sleep coaches" churned out by eight- to twelve-week programs that have no real authority to proclaim anything besides being the owner of a certificate suitable for framing. Crazy. I wonder if they have similar programs for people with no medical training who want to be infectious disease experts and treat their community's viral outbreaks? Or weekend orthopedic surgery programs.* If you end up not getting the advice you need on your child's sleep from this book, my suggestion is to evaluate the credentials of other sleep experts, specialists, or practitioners carefully before moving on.

Sleep coaching aside, when should an individual seek this kind of sleep health? The answer is *early*. Sleep problems have a way of starting small and slowly metastasizing to other aspects of our lives. Nipping your child's problems in the bud early can be a huge positive.

Making the decision to see a doctor is never easy, but you've made it through step one: understanding sleep doctors are out there and are available to see your child. What I mean is that many people don't realize that sleep specialists exist, and not only do they have medical training, but they also have years of specialized training in sleep. It is amusing how often parents ask me a variant of the question, "So are there really enough kids with sleep disorders for you to stay in business?"

Yes.

With your understanding of the existence of sleep doctors firmly in place, it is time to see one. While many sleep specialists/insurances do not require a referral, it is always a good idea to have one from your child's primary care doctor. In our clinic, we insist on communication with pediatricians. They often have loads of experience treating your child and valuable insights into their health. I consider them the quarterback of your child's health care (you, of course, are the coach). Getting a referral to a sleep specialist, in my opinion, should never be a problem. I tell parents all the time, if you ask for a sleep specialist referral for your child and her doctor refuses, get a new doctor. In my entire career, I have

---

* Like the woman who cut hair in her garage when you were growing up, just instead of hair, she's doing meniscus tears and ACLs.

never heard an argument against sitting down and talking to a sleep specialist that makes sense.

With the referral in place, it is time to pick a sleep specialist to see. Hopefully your child's clinician will have some helpful opinions as to who the best options would be given your child's specific issues. Keep in mind, as we spoke about before, "sleep specialist" can mean many different things. If we are assuming that your child is going to see a board-certified sleep specialist,* here are a few examples of the backgrounds to expect from the sleep MD you might see.

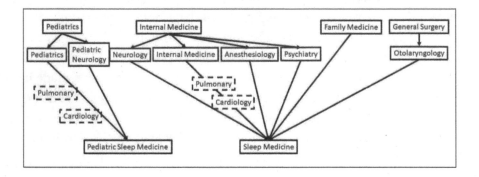

Neurologist

I am totally biased here, but to me, sleep is a discipline that falls squarely into neurology. Think about it. The state of being awake, vigilant, processing sensory information from the world around you is 100 percent brain, brain, brain. Similarly, the process of letting go of consciousness

---

* At the writing of this book, there are two different bodies that provide board certification for medical sleep specialists. The American Board of Sleep Medicine (ABSM) was the original sleep board certification. It stopped certifying physicians in 2006. I received my certification in September of 2005 . . . right before the doors closed! The second board is via the American Board of Medical Subspecialties. Either certification is fine. For the most part ABSM will be seen in older docs, the Sleep Medicine Certification Program in younger docs, and some docs like me just happened to come along at the precise time where we got snookered into paying to take both certification exams!

and transitioning into the sweet state of slumber is a brain process as well, full of chemicals, neurotransmitters, and minute electrical changes all geared toward maintaining the brain for optimal health and performance. Does anyone really want to argue this point?

To me, if your child seems to be struggling with issues related to sleep and their brains (associated seizures, terrible dreams, inattentiveness, restlessness in their legs, pain, etc.), I think dealing with a specialist versed in neurology is best.

Pediatrician

Okay, you've got me here. Sure, I will admit that a kid doctor is probably a good basis for a kid sleep specialist. Just keep in mind from the chart, the "pediatric sleep specialist" can be more tilted toward general pediatrics, pediatric pulmonary or cardiology, or neurology. Pediatric sleep specialists also tend to be fairly rare. In the United States, there are:

1.11 million physicians;

92,000 pediatricians;

18,000 neurologists, of which 900 are pediatric neurologists;

5,800 sleep specialists, of which . . .

270 are sleep pediatricians (.02 percent of all doctors).

Keep this in mind when you are searching for a sleep doc. There simply may not be a true pediatric sleep specialist available to you. Even I don't know that many!*

---

* Another thought about pediatrics. Do you know what the patient age range of a pediatrician generally encompasses? Birth to twenty-one years of age. I know this because when I was a neurology resident, and when things were slow in the emergency room, we would walk through the pediatric ER at the University of Virginia and see the "pediatric" exam rooms full of intoxicated "pediatric" patients. Strange to see a six-foot-one undergraduate student dressed in slacks and a blazer, moaning/ranting from a room with Minions painted on the wall. Good times.

The Pediatric Neurologist

I want to point out the real unicorn among the sleep specialists . . . the pediatric neurologist who is also trained in sleep medicine. Talk about rare! In a 2015 study, only 11 of 523 pediatric neurologists were boarded in sleep. That's 2 percent. That probably means there are about twenty of them out there . . . Even if there were forty, that would only represent 0.7 percent of all sleep specialists or 0.004 percent of all US physicians. To me, this person represents the ideal pediatric sleep physician, but their rarity makes them an almost magical creature.

Internal Medicine/Pulmonary Subspeciality

This is a typical sleep medicine specialist background because of one diagnosis: sleep apnea. If we look back in time, at some point an Australian pulmonologist became concerned enough about the nocturnal breathing of his patients to disassemble a Jacuzzi motor and glue it to his patient's face to help the patient breathe at night. This discovery and primitive treatment of sleep apnea exploded, and as with everything: follow the money.

a. Sleep apnea is a common disorder.

b. Fixing it helps people feel better, and we can charge for sleep studies and CPAP devices.

c. If we have a department full of people seeing patients, doing sleep studies and selling CPAPs, we can have an awesome end-of-the-year department party with those bacon-wrapped scallops.

d. The sleep division of the department of pulmonary medicine was born.

Even though I give my pulmonary brothers and sisters a hard time, there are some things that they are quite exceptional at: breathing disorders. While sleep has as much to do with the lungs as it does the gall bladder, breathing disturbances can wreck a night of sleep in a hurry, so if that seems to be your child's issue, the pulmonary doc (internist or pediatrician), might be a good place to start.

Psychiatrist/Psychologist

In the olden days of sleep medicine, you were quite likely to find a psychiatrist as a sleep specialist. I have had three amazing sleep mentors in my life: a pulmonologist, a neurologist, and a psychologist. Thinking about sleep and the psyche makes sense when you consider all the lore that surrounded dream interpretation and sleep. I was fortunate enough to know a researcher who did studies on couples in which he would give one partner a concrete item on which to concentrate hard when she went to bed. The other partner would go to bed concentrating hard on what he thought his partner was thinking about. The researcher wanted to know if the two individuals could "meet up" in their dreams and transmit real information. Whoa!*

To me, this might be the person to go to if your child has concurrent psychiatric issues like depression and anxiety, two conditions commonly seen in sleep clinics. While I think there is a danger sometimes with psychiatric professionals attributing all of a patient's symptoms to mood disturbance, often a sleep-trained psychiatrist or psychologist might be able to step back and differentiate the entities more effectively. I also think that within this group of sleep care providers, there is often a higher percentage of people trained in cognitive behavioral therapy for insomnia (CBT-I). CBT-I is without question the most effective treatment for insomnia, far better than the sleeping pills that most providers often want to throw at the condition.

---

* When I heard this, I spent several weeks trying my own experiment when my wife and I went to bed. Every night, I would concentrate on NASCAR, and in particular Dale Earnhardt Jr. (he was the only driver I was familiar with). I would picture his face, picture him driving, endorsing a Mountain Dew . . . all in the hopes that my wife would just spontaneously start talking about "Junior" one day, and how restrictor-plate racing was killing the joy of NASCAR races. So far, the experiment is yielding less than compelling results.

Otolaryngology, or Ear, Nose, Throat (ENT) Surgeon
In my opinion, these doctors are surgeons who are geared toward evaluating your kid for a surgical correction for their snoring, sleep apnea, or other breathing disturbance happening while they sleep.

General Internal Medicine/Family Medicine
Perfectly fine if you are seeing one of these folks, although outside of their broader fund of medical knowledge, I'm not sure what special gift they bring to the table, particularly when it comes to treating your child. If you are going the route of a generalist sleep specialist for your child, it would make sense to me to go see a generalist pediatrician who specializes in sleep, right?

Anesthesiologist (and Podiatrist, and Plastic Surgeon, and Immunologist, and Whatever Strange Specialty That Has a Few Sleep Specialists Within Its Ranks)
Let's just say sleep is cool, and I get why people would want to gravitate toward it. Just remember, sedation and sleep are really two different things. If your anesthesiologist is planning on sedating your child with propofol to get him to sleep, remember Michael Jackson, grab your child, and run away.

Time to Choose
There you go, a quick overview of the sleep specialists ready and excited to help you with your child. As you can see, when someone says "board-certified sleep doctor," it can mean a lot of things, not to mention the midlevels (nurse practitioners, physician assistants) who may work with these clinicians and provide potentially excellent care themselves. I have seen many a midlevel who seemed to be much more up-to-date on current sleep medicine research and treatment methods than the doctors for whom they work.

Do your research. Talk to your child's primary care provider. Be careful with putting too much emphasis on the online reviews of doctors. Being a sleep medicine doctor can be tough sometimes. Not only do we not have all the answers but also the answers we do have are sometimes not pleasing to parents.* I was told that one should never see a doctor with a perfect five-star review. It means she might be more concerned about pleasing patients rather than delivering quality care.

What to Expect from the Visit

Talking . . . lots of talking. In my opinion, what you have to say about your child is far more important than any test or sleep study that might be performed. What is the concern that you, your child, or your child's primary care doctor have in regards to his sleep or sleepiness during the day? How long has it been going on? What other aspects of your child's health seem to be involved? If he has been evaluated for sleep problems in the past, who was the provider and what information was discovered? Remember that even a "normal" or a "negative" test is helpful.

A quick word about sleep tests. On a daily basis, I am told that a child had a sleep study "a few years ago" but that "it didn't show anything" or that it was "normal because nobody ever mentioned it."

I have never in my career seen a sleep study that didn't tell me something useful.

Every sleep study shows something, and usually it shows a lot. It is not your fault that you don't know that; somebody probably neglected to go over it in detail with you. It is staggering how many parents bring me kids who have had sleep studies in the past but do not know what the report indicated. You and your insurance company probably paid several thousand dollars for that test. You deserve to know what it says about your child.†

One reason nobody went over the previous study is because it did not demonstrate the presence of sleep apnea. Awesome! That, however, is not the same thing as saying a sleep study is normal. How much did your

* I'm sorry that you think your five-year-old has never slept and needs a sedative to do so, but that's not how our clinic works.

† We often spend a significant amount of time in our clinic retroactively reviewing the studies of other doctors. It is all important and part of the story of your kid!

child sleep? How long did it take him to fall asleep? Did he show any signs of leg movements or dreaming? Sleep studies provide a wealth of information . . . even when they do not provide the answer as to what is wrong with your child.

One of the great things about being a specialist versus a primary care doctor is that I have the luxury of taking my time with your child.

That said, you must have copies of all these studies and bring them with you to see your sleep professional. Do not assume that something is unhelpful or unnecessary. Your sleep doctor will make that call.

Outside of taking a very thorough sleep and general medical history, in-person visits will often feature a brief examination. For some doctors (e.g., neurologists) the exam might be a bit more thorough than that done by the ENT, who just wants a look at your tonsils and throat.

After a thorough history and evaluation, it is time to make a plan. Don't be surprised if the plan involves more data collection on your part. Perhaps your doctors will want you to keep a detailed sleep journal of your child's sleeping patterns. If so, be as detailed as possible with the sleep log. In some cases, your doctor may want your child to wear a device that records information about his sleep over a longer period of time.

Sometimes, the initial interventions will be behavior modifications. Changing a napping schedule, adjusting a bedtime, or even increasing exercise or outdoor activity. Having read to this point in the book, you are no doubt an expert as to why your child's sleep specialist might make such recommendations.

The Sleep Study

There is a good chance that the evaluation of your child's sleep disturbance might include a sleep study. So far in the book, we have talked frequently about what a sleep study might tell us about your child's sleep, like how to interpret leg movements or differentiate breathing problems, but we have not really discussed what is involved with the actual night (or day) of testing.

Let me start by saying that it is entirely painless. I hear parents complain far more about the test than children because, yes, you guessed it, you'll be spending the night with them. While your child's accommodations will be comfortable, what you are sleeping on may not be as inviting. The current lab I'm affiliated with is in a hotel, so while your kid snoozes in her own queen-sized bed, you'll have your own immediately next to her. I have been in labs where Mom or Dad are relegated to a cot.

That said, kids generally have a good time. They can wear what they want, bring what they want, and are typically staying up a little later than normal watching cartoons while they are getting hooked up.

Kids are not dumb. They know the difference between the dentist's office and a candy shop. Their sleep study experience depends on many things, not the least of which is the interaction your child has with the sleep doctor. Kids at my clinic are greeted with fun children's books about sleep with titles like *The World Champion of Staying Awake* and *Goodnight Darth Vader* . . . you know, the classics. I don't wear a lab coat or bizarre bow tie. Just normal clothes. Trust needs to be established immediately. Don't want me to look at your tonsils? No problem, but I do have to wonder what you are hiding.

When I have decided that a sleep study is needed, rule number one is that I always ask the caregivers what they think about that idea and how well they think their child might handle it. I like to think that I can read your child after spending forty-five minutes together, but the simple fact of the matter is that there is one expert on your child in the exam room and it is *not* the middle-aged doctor who until recently thought a pony was just a small young horse.* If Mommy or Daddy think the idea of hooking wires up to their kid is going to end in tragedy and frustration, it is probably not going to happen.

If the study does happen, it will take place on some date in the future that is suitable to the parents' schedule. We focus a lot of attention on the kid's comfort during a sleep study. I also want to make sure Mom or Dad is comfortable too. You and your child will probably report to the lab around 6:00 to 7:00 p.m., shortly after dinner. Once settled, you will

* Sleep expert. Not equestrian expert, although for $995, I can take a thirty-five-hour course through the American Society of Equine Appraisers to become certified in appraising horses of all sizes . . . even ponies.

meet your technician for the night, and they should make you feel perfectly at home while preparing to get your child hooked up for the study (and maybe get your child's favorite stuffed animal hooked up too, if appropriate). Again, nothing hurts or should be uncomfortable or embarrassing.

Once hooked up, it is time to get into bed. If you need to lie down with your child, that's perfectly fine. If you want to read her some stories, I have some ideas! If your child is older, she may be eligible to stay by herself, or she may want you present. These items will all be worked out prior to the study.

If anything is needed during the night, the technician is always there, keeping an eye on the information that is being collected. I always tell patients that your technician will not only know your kid has woken up before you do, the tech will know before your child will. If any wire comes lose or if your child accidentally wets the bed, it is all perfectly fine. Your technician has seen it one hundred times and will know just what to do.

Generally, in the morning, the study is over and once your kid is disconnected from the wires, you can go home. I qualify this with "generally" because in some cases, you may be asked to stay for part of the next day with your kid to do a multiple sleep latency test (MSLT). An MSLT is a daytime nap study designed to evaluate your child for the presence of excessive daytime sleepiness.

The bottom line with sleep studies is that they are very easy and absolutely painless. They do, however, completely depend on your child feeling comfortable and relaxed. If your child is upset by the idea, or the situation causes him significant anxiety, it might be best to postpone the study for a while if possible. That time can be used to help alleviate anxieties, watch YouTube videos of "fun" sleep studies, and so on.

A word about sleep studies and kids. Most labs have rules about how old a child must be to spend the night unaccompanied. Typically, eighteen years old is the cutoff. Any age under the cutoff requires a parent to spend the night. Consider choosing the parent who relaxes the child the most and possibly snores the least, as many pediatric sleep studies often inadvertently lead to an adult sleep diagnosis.

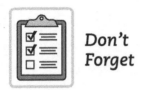 **Don't Forget**

1. Sleep specialists come from a variety of backgrounds and training, all eager to help your child sleep better.

2. Sleep studies are a valuable tool for learning more about the sleep of your child and any disturbances that may be affecting her.

Conclusion

You Made It. Given Today's Standards,
You May Be a Pediatric Sleep Expert.

I have been concerned for some time that when a parent walks through the parenting and self-help section in the bookstore, there is a message being sent from the bookshelves: make it through the first year or two and you have it made. It's as if sleep problems stop existing once a baby is sleeping through the night and starts eating food from a jar.

I think about kids and their sleep health constantly. I think just as much about the kids who never come to my clinic as the ones who do. I think about the young eighth grader in my wife's classroom who fell asleep every day without fail, and how often he got punished for the behavior.*

"He's got narcolepsy, I'm sure of it," she would say. Rules made it difficult to intervene medically, and all attempts to communicate with the student's mother were met with no replies. It pains me to hear about children with potentially solvable problems not getting the help, care, and education they require.

* Not by my wife. She was working to get him help!

And it matters. That boy was struggling academically, not because of inferior intellect or aptitude, but rather because of inferior sleep. Where could he have ended up had he been more rested and able to show what he knows? It's tragic to see students like this become adults and finally get their sleep situation fixed. There is often a thought that passes briefly though my mind: great, but what if?

In medicine, there are maladies that happen quickly, like a heart attack, and others that work slowly. In general, sleep disorders move slowly—they creep into our lives and make tiny changes. It's our job as parents to be especially vigilant, and always be questioning the sleep and rest of our kids. Once we are through the newborn and toddler years, we are not home free. Sleep needs to be treated and maintained like other foundational pieces in our children's health. Nutrition, exercise, mindfulness, and sleep are lifelong pillars to wellness. We want to prioritize and value them, but not stress over them.

Kids have more to think about today than ever before. The recent pandemic has created endless amounts of stress and uncertainty while at the same time eliminating protective social support systems. The stalwarts in place to keep sleep steady and on track, such as schools, religious institutions, and athletic events, have vanished for some individuals. Sleep quickly becomes the canary in the coal mine, with a disruption in sleep serving as an early sign that problems are occurring.

When I work with professional sports organizations, the first order of business is to establish a culture of communication when it comes to sleep. Forget the sleep trackers and in-depth assessments of sleep. Just create a space in which people can talk freely about their sleep, without judgment or consequence. In the same way, your children should be asked about their sleep frequently. Whenever possible, encourage them to share their feelings and concerns about their sleep.

One of the things I like about sleep problems is that they are usually fixable. Now you have the knowledge to get the process started for improving the sleep of your child, regardless of their age. Go forth with this newly found wisdom, engage meaningfully with your kid's teachers and doctors, and raise your healthy sleeper.

Appendix A

Laws of the House of Sleep*

1. Sleep always wins.
2. Perception of sleep and reality of sleep are two completely different things.
3. You can't fall asleep playing *Fortnite*.
4. Your kid couldn't "not sleep" even if he tried.
5. There is no such thing as a sleeping pill that doesn't lie.
6. Sleep hygiene alone is likely not going to fix your kid's sleep problem, but I hope it does.
7. You don't take your kid to the restaurant when she's not hungry, so don't put her to bed when she's not sleepy.
8. If you think your child is sleepy, but it takes him two hours to fall asleep, your child is not sleepy.
9. There are lots of things to be afraid of. Not sleeping is not one of them.
10. Not all kids stay up too late.
11. When your kid is fatigued, he should rest. When he is sleepy, he should go to bed. If he's going to bed when he's fatigued, there is a problem.
12. Do not assume your child's doctor knows anything about sleep.

* Apologies to Dr. Samuel Shem. I'm your biggest fan.

Children's Chronotype Questionnaire (CCTQ)

DEMOGRAPHICS

Please answer the following questions or choose the best answer.

Individual completing the questionnaire: ❑ Mother ❑ Father ❑ Other _____

Today's Date: ____/____/____ (day/month/year)

Child's Sex: ❑ Male ❑ Female

Child's Birth Date: ____/____/____ (day/month/year)

Child's Age: _____years

Child's Birth Order: _____

Is he/she an only child? ❑ Yes ❑ No

How many children are included in your nuclear family? _____

Do all children in your family have the same biological parents? ❑ Yes ❑ No

Child's current level of education: ❑ Preschool ❑ Kindergarten ❑ Grade _____
❑ Not attending school

If he/she attends school, how many days/week? _____

How many hours/day? _____

Does he/she go to day care or after-school care? ❑ Yes ❑ No

If yes, how many days a week? _____ How many hours/day? _____

Directions: The following questions ask about sleep/wake patterns during "Scheduled Days" in contrast to "Free Days." Think about your child's behavior during recent weeks when answering these questions. For questions with changing conditions (e.g., child goes to day care at 7:00 am 1 day/week and 9:00 am 3 days/week), fill in or select the most frequent or common answer.

SCHEDULED DAYS

Child's sleep-wake pattern is directly influenced by individual or family activities (e.g., by school, day care, work, athletics, etc.).

On Scheduled Days, my child . . .

1. . . . wakes up at _____:_____ am

2. . . . regularly wakes up: ❑ by him/herself ❑ with help from a family member ❑ with an alarm clock

3. . . . gets up at _____:_____ am

4. . . . is fully awake by_____:_____ am

5. . . . takes regular naps: ❏ Yes ❏ No

    If yes, he/she naps _____ days/week. If no, why does he/she not nap? _____

    _____

    _____

    If yes, he/she sleeps for _____ minutes/nap.

On nights before Scheduled Days . . .

6. . . . my child goes to bed (body in bed) at _____:_____ pm

7. . . . my child is ready to fall asleep (lights turned out) at _____:_____ pm

8. . . . it takes him/her _____ minutes to fall asleep (after lights turned out).

FREE DAYS

Child's sleep/wake pattern is "free" from the influence of individual or family activities (e.g., school, day care, work, athletics, etc.).

On Free Days, my child . . .

9. . . . normally wakes up at _____:_____ am

10. . . . wakes at his/her normal time on scheduled days, but then goes back to sleep after waking: ❏ Yes ❏ No

    If yes, my child goes back to sleep for ___ minutes after waking.

11. . . . gets up by _____:_____ am

12. . . . is fully awake by_____:_____ am

13. . . . takes regular naps: ❏ Yes ❏ No

    If yes, he/she naps _____ days per week. If no, why does he/she not nap? __

    _____

    If yes, he/she sleeps for _____ minutes per nap.

On nights before Free Days . . .

14. . . . my child goes to bed (body in bed) at _____:_____ pm

15. . . . my child is ready to fall asleep (lights turned out) at _____:_____ pm

16. . . . it takes him/her _____ minutes to fall asleep (after lights turned out).

Directions: For each of the following questions, please select the answer that best describes your child. Make your judgments based on how the behavior of your child was in recent weeks. There are no "right" or "wrong" answers.

17. *If your child has to be awakened, how difficult do you find it to wake your child up in the morning?
    (a) very difficult
    (b) fairly difficult
    (c) moderately difficult
    (d) slightly difficult
    (e) not at all difficult/my child never has to be awakened

18. *How alert is your child during the first half hour after having awakened in the morning?
    (a) not at all alert
    (b) slightly alert
    (c) moderately alert
    (d) fairly alert
    (e) very alert

19. Considering your child's "feeling best" rhythm, at what time would your child **get up** if he/she could decide by him/herself and if he/she were entirely free to plan the day (e.g., vacation)?
    (a) prior to 6:30 am
    (b) 6:30–7:14 am
    (c) 7:15–9:29 am
    (d) 9:30–10:14 am
    (e) after 10:15 am

20. Considering your child's "feeling best" rhythm, at what time would your child **go to bed** if he/she could decide by him/herself and if he/she were entirely free to plan the next day (e.g., weekend)?
    (a) prior to 6:59 pm
    (b) 7:00–7:59 pm
    (c) 8:00–9:59 pm
    (d) 10:00–10:59 pm
    (e) after 11:00 pm

21. Let's assume that your child has to be at peak performance for a test that will be mentally exhausting for 2 hours. Considering your child's "feeling best" rhythm and that you are entirely free to plan your child's day, which ONE of the three time intervals would you choose for the test?

    (a) 7:00–11:00 am

    (b) 11:00 am–3:00 pm

    (c) 3:00–8:00 pm

22. Let's assume that you have decided to enroll your child in an athletic activity (e.g., swimming). The only class available meets twice a week at 7 to 8 am. How do you think he/she will perform?

    (a) would be in very good form

    (b) would be in good form

    (c) would be in reasonable form

    (d) would find it difficult

    (e) would find it very difficult

23. At what time in the evening does your child seem tired and in need of sleep?

    (a) prior to 6:30 pm

    (b) 6:30–7:14 pm

    (c) 7:15–9:29 pm

    (d) 9:30–10:14pm

    (e) after 10:15 pm

24. *If your child had to get up every day at 6 am, what do you think it would be like for him/her?

    (a) very difficult

    (b) rather difficult

    (c) moderately difficult

    (d) a little difficult, but not a great problem

    (e) not at all difficult

25. *If your child always had to go to bed at _____, what do you think it would be like for him/her? (for 2 years old: 6:00 pm; for 2 to 4 years old: 6:30 pm; for 4 to 8 years old: 7:00 pm; for 8 to 11 years old: 7:30 pm)

    (a) very difficult

    (b) rather difficult

    (c) moderately difficult

(d) a little difficult, but not a great problem

(e) not at all difficult

26. When your child wakes up in the morning, how long does it take to be
fully awake?

(a) 0 minutes (i.e., immediately)

(b) 1 to 4 minutes

(c) 5 to 10 minutes

(d) 11 to 20 minutes

(e) ≥ 21 minutes

Directions: After answering the above questions, you may have a feeling which
"Chronotype" or "Time-of-Day Type" your child is. For example, if your child
would like to sleep quite a bit longer on "Free Days" compared to "Scheduled
Days" or if it is difficult for your child to get out of bed on Monday mornings, then
he/she is more likely to be an Evening Type person (a "Night Owl"). If your child,
however, regularly wakes up and feels perky once he/she gets out of bed, and your
child prefers to go to bed rather early than late, then he/she is more likely a Morning Type person (a "Morning Lark"). Please categorize your child using one of the
following choices. Please choose only one category!

27. My child is . . .

❒ definitely a Morning Type

❒ rather a Morning Type than an Evening Type

❒ neither a Morning nor an Evening Type

❒ rather an Evening Type than a Morning Type

❒ definitely an Evening Type

❒ I do not know

The M/E score is derived by adding points from answers 17–26 (a=1, b=2, c=3,
d=4, e=5), except as indicated by *, where point values have to be reversed.

PATIENT SLEEP LOG   **WEEK # ____**

Date	Example: 1/1/20							
Time in Bed	11:00 pm							
Time Asleep	12:30 am							
# of Awakenings	2							
Awakening Duration	5 min 30 min							
Awake for Good	6:15 am							
Out of Bed	7:30 am							
Napping	1 hour at 4pm							

Appendix B

Treatment Appendix

ADHD

Commonly utilized medications include:

FDA-APPROVED STIMULANTS

Adderall (50/50 mixture of dextroamphetamine and levoamphetamine)

dextroamphetamine (Dexedrine, DextroStat, Zenzedi) is a central nervous stimulant and enantiomer (molecular mirror) of levoamphetamine. It is a Schedule II controlled substance.

Evekeo (75 percent dextroamphetamine/25 percent levoamphetamine)

lisdexamfetamine (Vyvanse) is a psychomotor stimulant and amphetamine derivative. It is a Schedule II controlled substance.

methylphenidate (Ritalin, Concerta) is a psychomotor stimulant that acts as a norepinephrine/dopamine reuptake inhibitor. It is a Schedule II controlled substance.

mixed amphetamine salts (Adderall, Evekeo): These psychomotor stimulants are combinations of both enantiomers of the amphetamine molecule. The drugs vary based upon relative ratio of dextroamphetamine to levoamphetamine.

FDA-APPROVED NON-STIMULANTS

atomoxetine (Strattera) is a norepinephrine reuptake inhibitor used to treat ADHD in adults and children as young as six years old. It is not a controlled substance.

clonidine (Kapvay) is an alpha adrenergic receptor agonist used to treat a variety of conditions including ADHD. It is approved for children ages six to seventeen. It is not a controlled substance.

guanfacine (Tenex, Intuniv) is an α2A adrenergic receptor agonist used to treat ADHD in children ages six to seventeen. Intuniv is a long-acting version of Tenex. Guanfacine is not a controlled substance.

OFF-LABEL FDA-APPROVED DRUGS

modafinil (Provigil) has been used off-label in children with ADHD.

Narcolepsy

As of the writing of this book, there are basically seven different medications approved to treat the condition:

amphetamine (Adderall, Evekeo) is a psychomotor stimulant acting to increase norepinephrine and dopamine in the brain. Adderall is a 50/50 mixture of dextroamphetamine and levoamphetamine. A newer variant called Evekeo is a 75 percent dextroamphetamine and 25 percent levoamphetamine mixture, which may help minimize side effects of anxiety. These drugs are Schedule II controlled substances and are FDA approved for children as young as six years old.

armodafinil (NuVigil) has an unknown mechanism of action, but probably also acts as a selective, weak dopamine reuptake inhibitor. It is a Schedule IV controlled substance. Armodafinil is not approved for children and its effectiveness and safety in children under seventeen years old is not known.

methylphenidate (Ritalin) a psychomotor stimulant that acts as a norepinephrine/dopamine reuptake inhibitor. It is a Schedule II controlled substance.

modafinil (Provigil), like armodafinil, has a mechanism of action that is unknown, but probably acts as a selective, weak dopamine reuptake inhibitor. Like armodafinil, it is a Schedule IV controlled substance. Modafinil is not approved for children and its effectiveness and safety in children under seventeen years old is not known.

pitolisant (Wakix) is a selective histamine (H3) receptor antagonist/inverse agonist. We all know how antihistamines tend to cause sedation. Think of this drug as more of a pro-histamine drug, producing wakefulness. This drug was originally approved in Europe in 2016, and in the United States in late 2019, for the treatment of excessive daytime sleepiness. It was approved for the treatment of cataplexy in 2020. Currently, it is the only drug approved for narcolepsy that is not a controlled substance. Furthermore, the drug is only approved for patients eighteen years or older.

solriamfetol (Sunosi) is a wakefulness-promoting norepinephrine/dopamine reuptake inhibitor. It is approved for patients eighteen years or older, and like armodafinil/modafinil, it is a Schedule IV controlled substance.

Xyrem (sodium oxybate) has an unknown mechanism of action, but as a metabolite of GABA, it interacts with $GABA_B$ to facilitate wakefulness via dopamine and noradrenergic pathways. The drug is a Schedule III controlled substance and is FDA approved for children as young as seven years old.

Xywav (calcium, magnesium, potassium, and sodium oxybates) is a formulation of Xyrem, just approved in 2020, with approximately 90 percent less sodium. For a sense of this sodium reduction, the maximum dose of Xyrem (9 g nightly) contains 1640 mg of sodium (the American Heart Association recommends 1500 mg or less/day). The maximum dose of Xywav (also 9 g nightly) contains only 131 mg of sodium. The drug is a Schedule III controlled substance and is FDA approved for children as young as seven years old.

Currently, the only drugs approved for use in children are the stimulants (methylphenidate, amphetamine) and sodium oxybate, which is approved for kids as young as seven. It is not uncommon for the other medications to be used off-label in children; however, insurance coverage can be problematic.

Disclosure: I am a paid speaker and consultant for Jazz Pharmaceuticals (the maker of Xyrem, Xywav, and Sunosi) as well as Harmony

Bioscience (the maker of Wakix). In the past, I have been a speaker for both Provigil and Nuvigil.

Restless Legs Syndrome

As of the writing of this book, there are no medications approved to treat this condition in children. However, commonly utilized drugs include:

DOPAMINE AGONISTS
ropinirole (Requip) *FDA approved in adults
pramipexole (Mirapex) *FDA approved in adults

DOPIMANERGIC DRUGS
carbidopa/levodopa (Sinemet) *FDA approved in adults

BENZODIAZEPINES
clonazepam (Klonopin) *Schedule IV controlled substance

ALPHA-ADRENERGIC DRUGS
conidine (Catapres)

OTHER
gabapentin (Neurontin) *Schedule IV controlled substance

Enuresis

desmopressin (DDAVP) is an antidiuretic medication typically used for kids over the age of six.

oxybutynin (Ditropan) is an anticholinergic medication used for kids over the age of six.

imipramine (Tofranil) is a tricyclic antidepressant used to treat enuresis in kids over the age of six.

Acknowledgments

In the acknowledgments of my first book, I thanked my wife last. The process of writing that book was largely a stealthy endeavor with zero expectations. For this book, I feel like I leaned on you so much more. Wrapping up clinic and then disappearing to write placed terrific burdens on you, and your ability to shoulder them is why I am able to put this book out there. You are also a gifted editor, and I appreciate the time you spent reviewing my writing.

Thank you very much to Jeff Kleinman and Folio Literary Management for fighting to make this book a reality. You have a unique ability to listen, advise, and always remain optimistic.

To Lauren Appleton, I appreciate your time and enthusiasm for the project. Maybe *Tired AF* was not such a great idea for a book title.* Thanks to Alyssa Adler, Farin Schlussel, Victoria Adamo, and everyone at Avery for your dedication to this project.

Thanks to my clinic staff for your professionalism and ability to fill in the gaps I create when I'm getting pulled in several directions. The challenges of this year have been great. You have all stepped up and somehow made Charlottesville Neurology and Sleep Medicine a better experience for our patients (kids and adults).

* Yeah it was, come on.

Bibliography

References are organized in order of appearance.

Preface

Owens, Judith. "Classification and Epidemiology of Childhood Sleep Disorders." *Primary Care* 35, no. 3 (September 2008): 533–46.

Meltzer, Lisa J., Melissa R. Plaufcan, Jocelyn H. Thomas, and Jodi A. Mindell. "Sleep Problems and Sleep Disorders in Pediatric Primary Care: Treatment Recommendations, Persistence, and Health Care Utilization." *Journal of Clinical Sleep Medicine* 10, no. 4 (April 2014): 421–26.

Van Dyk, Tori R., Stephen P. Becker, and Kelly C. Byars. "Rates of Mental Health Symptoms and Associations with Self-Reported Sleep Quality and Sleep Hygiene in Adolescents Presenting for Insomnia Treatment." *Journal of Clinical Sleep Medicine* 15, no. 10 (October 2019): 1433–42.

Marsh, Sarah. "Children's Lack of Sleep Is 'Hidden Health Crisis,' Experts Say." *Guardian*, September 30, 2018, https://www.theguardian.com/lifeandstyle /2018/sep/30/childrens-lack-of-sleep-is-hidden-health-crisis-experts-say.

Mindell, Jodi, Mary Carskadon, Ronald Chervin, and Lisa Meltzer. "2004 Sleep in America Poll." Washington, DC: National Sleep Foundation, 2004.

Centers for Disease Control and Prevention. "National Diabetes Statistics Report, 2020." Atlanta: Centers for Disease Control and Prevention, US Department of Health and Human Services, 2020.

Danielson, Melissa L., Rebecca H. Bitsko, Reem M. Ghandour, Joseph R. Holbrook, Michael D. Kogan, and Stephen J. Blumberg. "Prevalence of Parent-Reported ADHD Diagnosis and Associated Treatment Among US Children and Adolescents, 2016." *Journal of Clinical Child and Adolescent Psychology* 47, no. 2 (March–April 2018): 199–212.

Thapar, Anita, Stephan Collishaw, Daniel S. Pine, and Ajay K. Thapar. "Depression in Adolescence." *Lancet* 379, no. 9820 (March 17, 2012): 1056–67.

Hales, Craig M., Margaret D. Carroll, Cheryl D. Fryar, and Cynthia L. Ogden. "Prevalence of Obesity Among Adults and Youth: United States, 2015–2016." NCHS Data Brief, no. 288. National Center for Health Statistics, 2017.

Winsler, Adam, Aaron Deutsch, Robert Daniel Vorona, Phyllis Abramczyk Payne, and Mariana Szklo-Coxe. "Sleepless in Fairfax: The Difference One More Hour of Sleep Can Make for Teen Hopelessness, Suicidal Ideation, and Substance Use." *Journal of Youth Adolescence* 44, no. 2 (February 2015): 362–78.

Introduction

Richardson, Anne Steese. *Better Babies and Their Care*. New York: Frederick A. Stokes, 2014.

Chapter 1: Sleep 101 for Parents:
How Sleep Works in Your Kid's Brain

Rurak, Dan. "Fetal Sleep and Spontaneous Behavior in Utero: Animal and Clinical Studies." In *Prenatal and Postnatal Determinants of Development*, edited by David W. Walker, 89–146. Melbourne: Humana Press, 2016.

Ciarleglio, Christopher M., John C. Axley, Benjamin R. Strauss, Karen L. Gamble, and Douglas G. McMahon. "Perinatal Photoperiod Imprints the Circadian Clock." *Nature Neuroscience* 14 (2011): 25–27.

Lecanuet, Jean-Pierre, and Anne-Yvonne Jacquet. "Fetal Responsiveness to Maternal Passive Swinging in Low Heart Rate Variability State: Effects of Stimulation Direction and Duration." *Developmental Psychobiology* 40, no. 1 (January 2002): 57–67.

Nakajima, Yukari, Kenji Yamaji, and Kazutomo Ohashi. "Fetal Heart Rate and Uterine Contraction During Automobile Driving." *Journal of Obstetrics and Gynaecology Research* 30, no. 1 (February 2004): 15–19.

Hoppenbrouwers, Toke, Diane Combs, Juan Carlos Ugartechea, Joan Hodgman, M. B. Sterman, and R. M. Harper. "Fetal Heart Rates During Maternal Wakefulness and Sleep." *Obstetrics Gynecology* 57, no. 3 (March 1981): 301–9.

Patrick, J. K. Campbell, L. Carmichael, and C. Probert. "Influence of Maternal Heart Rate and Gross Fetal Body Movements on the Daily Pattern of Fetal Heart Rate Near Term." *American Journal of Obstetrics Gynecology* 144, no. 5 (November 1982): 533–38.

Richardson, Anne Steese. *Better Babies and Their Care*. New York: Frederick A. Stokes, 1914.

Uchida, Mariko O., Takeshi Arimitsu, Kiyomi Yatabe, Kazushige Ikeda, Takao Takahashi, and Yasuyo Minagawa. "Effect of Mother's Voice on Neonatal Respiratory Activity and EEG Delta Amplitude." *Developmental Psychobiology* 60, no. 2 (March 2018): 140–49.

Shellhaas, Renée A., Joseph W. Burns, John D. E. Barks, Fauziya Hassan F, and Ronald D. Chervin. "Maternal Voice and Infant Sleep in the Neonatal Intensive Care Unit." *Pediatrics* 144, no. 3 (September 2019): e20190288.

Eisermann, Monika, Anna Kaminska, Marie-Laure Moutard, C. Soufflet, and Perrine Plouin. "Normal EEG in Childhood: From Neonates to Adolescents." *Neurophysiologie Clinique* 43, no. 1 (January 2013): 35–65.

Hirshkowitz, Max, Kaitlyn Whiton, Steven M. Albert, Cathy Alessi, Oliviero Bruni, Lydia DonCarlos, Nancy Hazen, John Herman, Eliot S. Katz, Leila Kheirandish-Gozal, David N. Neubauer, Anne E. O'Donnell, Maurice Ohayon, John Peever, Robert Rawding, Ramesh C. Sachdeva, Belinda Setters, Michael V. Vitiello, J. Catesby Ware, and Paula J. Adams Hillard. "National Sleep Foundation's Sleep Time Duration Recommendations: Methodology and Results Summary." *Sleep Health* 1, no. 1 (March 2015): 40-43.

Henderson, Jacqueline M., Karyn G. France, Joseph L. Owens, and Neville M. Blampied. "Sleeping Through the Night: The Consolidation of Self-Regulated Sleep Across the First Year of Life." *Pediatrics* 126, no. 5 (November 2010): e1081–87.

Chapter 2: Sleep Beliefs: *Your Parents Were Wrong About Everything, from Pills to Naps to Cosleeping.*

Eley, Thalia C., Tom A. McAdams, Fruhling V. Rijsdijk, Paul Lichtenstein, Jurgita Narusyte, David Reiss, Erica L. Spotts, Jody M. Ganiban, and Jenae M. Neiderhiser. "The Intergenerational Transmission of Anxiety: A Children-of-Twins Study." *American Journal of Psychiatry* 172, no. 7 (July 2015): 630–37.

Schmidt, Megan. "Short Sleeper 'Syndrome': When You Can Get By on Just a Few Hours of Sleep." *Discover*, September 20, 2019, https://www.discovermagazine.com/health/short-sleeper-syndrome-when-you-can-get-by-on-just-a-few-hours-of-sleep.

Knutson, Kristen L., Eve Van Cauter, Paul J. Rathouz, Thomas DeLeire, and Diane S. Lauderdale. "Trends in the Prevalence of Short Sleepers in the USA: 1975–2006." *Sleep* 33, no. 1 (January 2010): 37–45.

Richardson, Anne Steese. *Better Babies and Their Care.* New York: Frederick A. Stokes, 1914.

Murphy, Sherry L., Jiaquan Xu, Kenneth D. Kochanek, and Elizabeth Arias. "Mortality in the United States, 2017." NCHS Data Brief, no. 328. Hyattsville, MD: National Center for Health Statistics. 2018.

Goldstein, Richard D., Peter S. Blair, Mary Ann Sens, Carrie K. Shapiro-Mendoza, Henry F. Krous, Torleiv O. Rognum, and Rachel Y. Moon. "Inconsistent Classification of Unexplained Sudden Deaths in Infants and Children Hinders Surveillance, Prevention and Research: Recommendations from the 3rd

International Congress on Sudden Infant and Child Death." *Forensic Science, Medicine, and Pathology* 15, no. 4 (December 2019): 622–28.

Moon, Rachel Y. "SIDS and Other Sleep-Related Infant Deaths: Updated 2016 Recommendations for a Safe Infant Sleeping Environment." *Pediatrics* 138, no. 5 (November 2016): e20162940.

Blair, Peter S., Peter John Fleming, I. J. Smith, Martin Ward Platt, Jeanine Young, P. Nadin, P. J. Berry, and Jean Golding. "Babies Sleeping with Parents: Case-Control Study of Factors Influencing the Risk of the Sudden Infant Death Syndrome. CESDI SUDI Research Group." *BMJ* 319, no. 7233 (December 4, 1999): 1457–61.

Blair, Peter S., Peter Sidebotham, Carol Evason-Coombe, Margaret Edmonds, Elen M. A. Heckstall-Smith, and Peter Fleming. "Hazardous Cosleeping Environments and Risk Factors Amenable to Change: Case-Control Study of SIDS in South West England." *BMJ* (October 13, 2009): 339:b3666.

McKenna, James J. *Safe Infant Sleep; Expert Answers to Your Cosleeping Questions.* Washington, DC: Platypus Media, 2020.

———. "Safe Cosleeping Guidelines." University of Notre Dame Mother-Baby Behavioral Sleep Laboratory, accessed April 29, 2021, https://cosleeping.nd.edu /safe-co-sleeping-guidelines/.

Cortesi, Flavia, Flavia Giannotti, Teresa Sebastiani, Cristina Vagnoni, and Patrizia Marioni. "Cosleeping Versus Solitary Sleeping in Children with Bedtime Problems: Child Emotional Problems and Parental Distress." *Behavioral Sleep Medicine* 6, no. 2 (2008): 89–105.

McCarthy, Fergus P., Linda M. O'Keeffe, Ali S. Khashan, Robyn A. North, Lucilla Poston, Lesley M. E. McCowan, Philip N. Baker, Gus A. Dekker, Claire T. Roberts, James J. Walker, and Louise C. Kenny. "Association Between Maternal Alcohol Consumption in Early Pregnancy and Pregnancy Outcomes." *Obstetrics & Gynecology* 122, no. 4 (October 2013): 830–37.

Liu, Jianghong, Rui Feng, Xiaopeng Ji, Naixue Cui, Adrian Raine, and Sara C. Mednick. "Midday Napping in Children: Associations Between Nap Frequency and Duration Across Cognitive, Positive Psychological Well-Being, Behavioral, and Metabolic Health Outcomes." *Sleep* 42, no. 9 (September 6, 2019): zsz126.

Horváth, Klára, and Kim Plunkett. "Spotlight on Daytime Napping During Early Childhood." *Nature and Science of Sleep* 10 (March 9, 2018): 97–104.

Lam, Janet C., E. Mark Mahone, Thornton Mason, and Steven M. Scharf. "The Effects of Napping on Cognitive Function in Preschoolers." *Journal of Developmental & Behavioral Pediatrics* 32, no. 2 (February–March 2011): 90–97.

Hofer-Tinguely, Gilberte, Peter Achermann, Hans-Peter Landolt, Sabine J. Regel, Julia V. Rétey, Roland Dürr, Alexander A. Borbély, and Julie M. Gottselig. "Sleep Inertia: Performance Changes After Sleep, Rest and Active Waking." *Brain Research. Cognitive Brain Research* 22, no. 3 (March 2005): 323–31.

Mednick, Sara C, Tal Makovski, Denise J. Cai, and Y. V. Jiang. "Sleep and Rest Facilitate Implicit Memory in a Visual Search Task." *Vision Research* 49, no. 21 (October 2009): 2557–65.

Erland, Lauren A., and Praveen K. Saxena. "Melatonin Natural Health Products and Supplements: Presence of Serotonin and Significant Variability of Melatonin Content." *Journal of Clinical Sleep Medicine* 13, no. 2 (February 15, 2017): 275–81.

Chapter 3: Pediatric Insomnia: *Understanding What It Means When Your Child Says He "Can't Sleep"*

Richardson, Anna Steese. *Little Talks on Babyology: Sleep*. New York: Woman's Home Companion, 1913.

Bock, Dirk E., Elizabeth Roach-Fox, Jamie A. Seabrook, Michael J. Rieder, and Doreen Matsui. "Sleep-Promoting Medications in Children: Physician Prescribing Habits in Southwestern Ontario, Canada." *Sleep Med* 17 (January 2016): 52–56.

Chapter 4: Sleep Schedules: *A Scheduled Child Makes a Happy Parent.*

Richardson, Anne Steese. *Better Babies and Their Care*. New York: Frederick A. Stokes, 1914.

McPhail, S., V. Vleck, A. Herk-Heimer, and Z. Herk-Heimer. "Privacy and Ethical Concerns Regarding the Mass Collection of Sleep Data via Audio-Telly-O-Tally-O Count Device." *Sleep* (1962): 900–03.

Narvaez, Darcia F. "Dangers of 'Crying It Out': The Practice Comes from Comes from [*sic*] a Misunderstanding of Child Development." *Psychology Today*, December 11, 2011, https://www.psychologytoday.com/us/blog/moral-landscapes/201112/dangers-crying-it-out#:~:text=This20expands%20to%20other%20caregivers,Babies%20grow%20from%20being%20held.

Chapter 5: Insufficient-Sleep Disorders and School Start Times: *How to Find a School Bus in the Dark*

Tsao, Hoi See, Annie Gjelsvik, Sakina Sojar, and Siraj Amanullah. "Sounding the Alarm on the Importance of Sleep: The Negative Impact of Insufficient Sleep on Childhood Flourishing." *Pediatrics* 146, meeting abstract (2020): 49–50.

Wheaton, Anne G., Sherry Everett Jones, Adina C. Cooper, and Janet B. Croft. "Short Sleep Duration Among Middle School and High School Students—United States, 2015." *Morbidity and Mortality Weekly Report* 67, no. 3 (January 26, 2018): 85–90.

Richardson, Anne Steese. *Better Babies and Their Care*. New York: Frederick A. Stokes, 1914.

Sadeh, Avi. "Consequences of Sleep Loss or Sleep Disruption in Children." *Sleep Medicine Clinics* 2, no. 3 (September 2007): 513–20.

Janssen, Kitty C., Sivanes Phillipson, Justen O'Connor, and Murray W. Johns. "Validation of the Epworth Sleepiness Scale for Children and Adolescents Using Rasch Analysis." *Sleep Medicine* 33 (May 2017): 30–35.

Rudd, Brittany N., Amy Holtzworth-Munroe, Brian M. D'Onofrio, and Mary Waldron. "Parental Relationship Dissolution and Child Development: The Role of Child Sleep Quality." *Sleep* 42, no. 2 (February 1, 2019): zsy224.

Twenge, Jean M., Garrett C. Hisler, and Zlatan Krizan. "Associations Between Screen Time and Sleep Duration Are Primarily Driven by Portable Electronic Devices: Evidence from a Population-Based Study of U.S. Children Ages 0–17." *Sleep Medicine* 56 (April 2019): 211–18.

Hopkins, Bobbi. "Is the Pandemic Having an Impact on the Way Children Sleep?" Johns Hopkins All Children's Hospital Newsroom, April 27, 2020, https://www.hopkinsallchildrens.org/ACH-News/General-News/Is--the-Pandemic-Having-an-Impact-on-the-Way-Childr.

Jacob, Brian A., and Jonah E. Rockoff. "Organizing Schools to Improve Student Achievement: Start Times, Grade Configurations, and Teacher Assignments." Hamilton Project, September 27, 2011, https://www.hamiltonproject.org/papers/organizing_schools_to_improve_student_achievement_start_times_grade_co.

Carrell, Scott E., Teny Maghakian, and James E. West. "A's from Zzzz's? The Causal Effect of School Start Time on the Academic Achievement of Adolescents." *American Economic Journal: Economic Policy* 3, no. 3 (August 2011): 62–81.

Shi, Guangsen, Lijuan Xing, David Wu, Bula J. Bhattacharyya, Christopher R. Jones, Thomas McMahon, S. Y. Christin Chong, Jason A. Chen, Giovanni Coppola, Daniel Geschwind, Andrew Krystal, Louis J. Ptáček, and Ying-Hui Fu. "A Rare Mutation of β_1-Adrenergic Receptor Affects Sleep/Wake Behaviors." *Neuron* 103, no. 6 (September 2019): 1044–55.e7.

Åkerstedt, Torbjörn, Francesca Ghilotti, Alessandra Grotta, Hongwei Zhao, Hans-Olov Adami, Ylva Trolle-Lagerros, and Rino Bellocco. "Sleep Duration and Mortality—Does Weekend Sleep Matter?" *Journal of Sleep Research* 28, no. 1 (February 2019): e12712.

Chapter 6: Sleep and Disorders of Attention:
"Can You Repeat That? I Was Thinking About a Spaceship."

Lange, Klaus W., Susanne Reichl, Katharina M. Lange, Lara Tucha, and Oliver Tucha. "The History of Attention Deficit Hyperactivity Disorder." *Attention Deficit and Hyperactivity Disorders* 2, no. 4 (2010): 241–55.

Tso, Winnie, Meanne Chan, Frederick K. Ho, Nirmala Rao, Albert M. Li, Ko Ling Chan, Agnes Tiwari, Ian C. K. Wong, Yun Kwok Wing, Benjamin Van Voorhees,

Sophia Ling Li, Winnie H. S. Goh, and Patrick Ip. "Early Sleep Deprivation and Attention-Deficit/Hyperactivity Disorder." *Pediatric Research* 85, no. 4 (March 2019): 449–55.

Kirov, Roumen, Joerg Kinkelbur, Susanne Heipke, Tatiana Kostanecka-Endress, Moritz Westhoff, Stefan Cohrs, Eckart Ruther, Goran Hajak, Tobias Banaschewski, and Aribert Rothenberger. "Is There a Specific Polysomnographic Sleep Pattern in Children with Attention Deficit/Hyperactivity Disorder?" *Journal of Sleep Research* 13, no. 1 (March 2004): 87–93.

Owens, Judith A., Rolanda Maxim, Chantelle Nobile, Melissa McGuinn, and Michael Msall. "Parental and Self-Report of Sleep in Children with Attention-Deficit/Hyperactivity Disorder." *Archives of Pediatrics & Adolescent Medicine* 154, no. 6 (June 2000): 549–55.

Scott, Nicola, Peter S. Blair, Alan M. Emond, Peter J. Fleming, Joanna S. Humphreys, John Henderson, and Paul Gringras. "Sleep Patterns in Children with ADHD: A Population-Based Cohort Study from Birth to 11 Years." *Journal of Sleep Research* 22, no. 2 (April 2013): 121–28.

Lecendreux, Michel, Eric Konofal, Manuel Bouvard, Bruno Falissard, and Marie-Christine Mouren-Siméoni. "Sleep and Alertness in Children with ADHD." *Journal of Child Psychology and Psychiatry* 41, no. 6 (September 2000): 803–12.

Centers for Disease Control and Prevention. "ADHD Throughout the Years." Atlanta: Centers for Disease Control and Prevention, US Department of Health and Human Services; 2020, https://www.cdc.gov/ncbddd/adhd/timeline.html.

Ra, Chaelin K., Junhan Cho, Matthew Stone, Julianne De La Cerda, Nicholas I. Goldenson, Elizabeth Moroney, Irene Tung, Steve S. Lee, and Adam M. Leventhal. "Association of Digital Media Use with Subsequent Symptoms of Attention-Deficit/Hyperactivity Disorder Among Adolescents." *JAMA* 320, no. 3 (July 2018): 255–63.

Bijlenga, Denise, Madelon A. Vollebregt, J. J. Sandra Kooij, and Martijn Arns. "The Role of the Circadian System in the Etiology and Pathophysiology of ADHD: Time to Redefine ADHD?" *Attention Deficit and Hyperactivity Disorders* 11, no. 1 (March 2019): 5–19.

Shur-Fen Gau, Susan. "Prevalence of Sleep Problems and Their Association with Inattention/Hyperactivity Among Children Aged 6–15 in Taiwan." *Journal of Sleep Research* 15, no. 4 (December 2006): 403–14.

Hvolby, Allan. "Associations of Sleep Disturbance with ADHD: Implications for Treatment." *Attention Deficit and Hyperactivity Disorders* 7, no. 1 (March 2015): 1–18.

Corkum, Penny, Rosemary Tannick, and Harvey Moldofsky. "Sleep Disturbances in Children with Attention-Deficit/Hyperactivity Disorder." *Journal of American Academy of Child and Adolescent Psychiatry* 37, no. 6 (June 1998): 637–46.

Yoon, Sun Young Rosalia, Umesh Jain, and Colin Shapiro. "Sleep in Attention-Deficit/Hyperactivity Disorder in Children and Adults: Past, Present, and Future." *Sleep Medicine Reviews* 16, no. 4 (August 2012): 371–88.

Rybak, Yuri E., Heather E. McNeely, Bronwyn E. Mackenzie, Umesh R. Jain, and Robert D. Levitan. "An Open Trial of Light Therapy in Adult Attention-Deficit/Hyperactivity Disorder." *Journal of Clinical Psychiatry* 67, no. 10 (October 2006): 1527–35.

Sciberras, Emma, Melissa Mulraney, Fiona Mensah, F. Oberklaid, D. Efron, and Harriet Hiscock. "Sustained Impact of a Sleep Intervention and Moderators of Treatment Outcome for Children with ADHD: A Randomised Controlled Trial." *Psychological Medicine* 50, no. 2 (January 2020): 210–19.

Kozielec, T., and B. Starobrat-Hermelin. "Assessment of Magnesium Levels in Children with Attention Deficit Hyperactivity Disorder (ADHD)." *Magnesium Research* 10, no. 2 (June 1997): 143–48.

Skalny, Anatoly V., Anna L. Mazaletskaya, Olga P. Ajsuvakova, Geir Bjørklund, Margarita G. Skalnaya, Lyubov N. Chernova, Andrey A. Skalny, and Alexey A. Tinkov. "Magnesium Status in Children with Attention-Deficit/Hyperactivity Disorder and/or Autism Spectrum Disorder." *Journal of the Korean Academy of Child and Adolescent Psychiatry* 31, no. 1 (January 2020): 41–45.

Effatpanah, Mohammad, Farzaneh Motamed, Mehri Najafi, Fatemeh Farahmand, Gholamhosein Fallahi, Davood Motaharizad, Mir Saeed Yekaninejad, Mostafa Qorbani, and Jayran Zebardast. "Prevalence of Attention Deficit Hyperactivity Disorder in Pediatrics Patients Newly Diagnosed with Gastroesophageal Reflux Disease." *Internet Journal of Pediatrics and Neonatology* 5, no. 9: 5609–16.

Turner, Danielle. "A Review of the Use of Modafinil for Attention-Deficit Hyperactivity Disorder." *Expert Review of Neurotherapeutics* 6, no. 4 (April 2006): 455–68.

Chapter 7: Narcolepsy: *"Given How Much Your Child Sleeps in My Class, This C+ Is a Remarkable Achievement."*

Sarkanen, Tomi, Anniina Alakuijala, Ilkka Julkunen, and Markku Partinen. "Narcolepsy Associated with Pandemrix Vaccine." *Current Neurology and Neuroscience Reports* 18, no. 7 (June 2018): 43.

Thorpy, Michael J., and Ana C. Krieger. "Delayed Diagnosis of Narcolepsy: Characterization and Impact." *Sleep Medicine* 15, no. 5 (May 2014): 502–07.

Carter, Lawrence P., Christine Acebo, and Ann Kim. "Patients' Journeys to a Narcolepsy Diagnosis: A Physician Survey and Retrospective Chart Review." *Postgraduate Medical Journal* 126, no. 3 (May 2014): 216–24.

Nevsimalova, Sona. "Narcolepsy in Childhood." *Sleep Medicine Reviews* 13, no. 2 (April 2009): 169–80.

Karjalainen, Satu, Anna-Maria Nyrhilä, Kaarina Määttä, and Satu Uusiautti. "Going to School with Narcolepsy—Perceptions of Families and Teachers of Children with Narcolepsy." *Early Child Development and Care* 184, no. 6 (August 2013): 869–81.

Rosenberg, Russell, and Ann Y. Kim. "The AWAKEN Survey: Knowledge of Narcolepsy Among Physicians and the General Population." *Postgraduate Medicine Journal* 126, no. 1 (January 2014): 78–86.

Chapter 8: Circadian Issues in Children and Teenagers:
"Good Morning, Mom. What's for Dinner?"

Macnish, Robert. *The Philosophy of Sleep.* New York: Appleton, 1834.

Richardson, Anne Steese. *Better Babies and Their Care.* New York: Frederick A. Stokes, 1914.

Cheng, Feng-Li, Yun-Fang An, Zhuo-Qin Han, Chao Li, Ze-Qing Li, Ping-Chang Yang, and Chang-Qing Zhao. "*Period2* Gene Regulates Diurnal Changes of Nasal Symptoms in an Allergic Rhinitis Mouse Model." *International Forum of Allergy and Rhinology* 10, no. 11 (November 2020): 1236–48.

Aschoff, Jürgen. "Circadian Rhythms in Man." *Science* 148, no 3676 (June 11, 1965): 1427–32.

American Academy of Sleep Medicine. *International Classification of Sleep Disorders,* 3rd ed. Darien, IL, 2014.

Sivertsen, Bø, Allison G. Harvey, Ståle Pallesen, and Mari Hysing. "Mental Health Problems in Adolescents with Delayed Sleep Phase: Results from a Large Population-Based Study in Norway." *Journal of Sleep Research* 24, no. 1 (February 2015): 11–18.

Werner, Helene, Monique K. Lebourgeois, Anja Geiger, and Oskar G. Jenni. "Assessment of Chronotype in Four- to Eleven-Year-Old Children: Reliability and Validity of the Children's Chronotype Questionnaire (CCTQ)." *Chronobiology International* 26, no. 5 (July 2009): 992–1014.

Chapter 9: Technology and Children: *"There Will Be No Television Until You Finish That Homework on Your iPad!"*

Murray, John P. "Television and Violence: Implications of the Surgeon General's Research Program." *American Psychologist* 28, no. 6 (1973): 472–78.

Comtet, Henri, Pierre A. Geoffroy, Mio Kobayashi Frisk, Jeffrey Hubbard, Ludivine Robin-Choteau, Laurent Calvel, Laurence Hugueny, Antoine U. Viola, and Patrice Bourgin. "Light Therapy with Boxes or Glasses to Counteract Effects of Acute Sleep Deprivation." *Scientific Reports* 9, no. 1 (December 2019): 18073.

Cho, Chul-Hyun, Ho-Kyoung Yoon, Seung-Gul Kang, Leen Kim, Eun-Il Lee, and Heon-Jeong Lee. "Impact of Exposure to Dim Light at Night on Sleep in Female and Comparison with Male Subjects." *Psychiatry Investigation* 15, no. 5 (May 2018): 520–30.

Mouland, Joshua W., Franck Martial, Alex Watson, Robert J. Lucas, and Timothy M. Brown. "Cones Support Alignment to an Inconsistent World by Suppressing Mouse Circadian Responses to the Blue Colors Associated with Twilight." *Current Biology* 29, no. 24 (December 16, 2019): 4260–67.e4.

Hale, Lauren, and Stanford Guan. "Screen Time and Sleep Among School-Aged Children and Adolescents: A Systematic Literature Review." *Sleep Medicine Reviews* 21 (June 2015): 50–58.

Ivory, James D., and Sriram Kalyanaraman. "The Effects of Technological Advancement and Violent Content in Video Games on Players' Feelings of Presence, Involvement, Physiological Arousal, and Aggression." *Journal of Communication* 57, no. 3 (September 2007): 532–55.

Chapter 10: Nightmares, Night Terrors, Sleepwalking and -talking and -eating: *More Nighttime Drama and Screaming than a* Real Housewives *Episode*

American Academy of Sleep Medicine. International classification of sleep disorders, 3rd ed. Darien, IL. 2014.

Carter, Kevin A., Nathanael E. Hathaway, and Christine F. Lettieri. "Common Sleep Disorders in Children." *American Family Physician* 89, no. 5 (March 2014): 368–77.

Challamel, M. J. "La somniloquie [Sleep talking]." *Revue Neurologique* (Paris) 157, no. 11, pt. 2 (November 2001): S112–14.

Laberge, Luc, Richard E. Tremblay, Frank Vitaro, and Jacques Montplaisir. "Development of Parasomnias from Childhood to Early Adolescence." *Pediatrics* 106, no. 1, (July 2000): 67–74.

Arnulf, Isabelle. "Sleepwalking." *Current Biology* 28, no. 22 (November 2018): R1288–89.

Petit, Dominique, Marie-Hélène Pennestri, Jean Paquet, Alex Desautels, Antonio Zadra, Frank Vitaro, Richard E. Tremblay, Michel Boivin, and Jacques Montplaisir. "Childhood Sleepwalking and Sleep Terrors: A Longitudinal Study of Prevalence and Familial Aggregation." *JAMA Pediatrics* 169, no. 7 (July 2015): 653–58.

Stallman, Helen M., and Mark Kohler. "Prevalence of Sleepwalking: A Systematic Review and Meta-Analysis." *PLoS One* 11, no. 11 (November 10, 2016): e0164769.

Foster, Josh, Alexis Mauger, Katie Thomasson, Stephanie White, and Lee Taylor. "Effect of Acetaminophen Ingestion on Thermoregulation of Normothermic, Non-Febrile Humans." *Frontiers in Pharmacology* 7 (March 14, 2016): 54.

Winkelman, John W. "Clinical and Polysomnographic Features of Sleep-Related Eating Disorder." *Journal of Clinical Psychiatry* 59, no. 1 (January 1998): 14–19.

———. "Treatment of Nocturnal Eating Syndrome and Sleep-Related Eating Disorder with Topiramate." *Sleep Medicine* 4, no. 3 (May 2003): 243–46.

Machado, Eduardo, Cibele Dal-Fabbro, Paulo Alfonson Cunali, and Osvaldo Bazzan Kaizer. "Prevalence of Sleep Bruxism in Children: A Systematic Review." *Dental Press Journal of Orthodontics* 19, no. 6 (November–December 2014): 54–61.

Tachibana, Masaya, Takafumi Kato, Kumi Kato-Nishimura, Shigeyuki Matsuzawa, Ikuko Mohri, and Masako Taniike. "Associations of Sleep Bruxism with Age, Sleep Apnea, and Daytime Problematic Behaviors in Children." *Oral Diseases* 22, no. 6 (September 2016): 557–65.

Oksenberg, Arie, and Elena Arons. "Sleep Bruxism Related to Obstructive Sleep Apnea: The Effect of Continuous Positive Airway Pressure." *Sleep Medicine* 3, no. 6 (November 2002): 513–15.

Oliveira, Marcelo Tomás de, Sandra Teixeira Bittencourt, Karina Marcon, Samia Destro, and Jefferson Ricardo Pereira. "Sleep Bruxism and Anxiety Level in Children." *Brazilian Oral Research* 29 (January 2015): 1–5.

Li, Yuanyuan, Fan Yu, Lina Niu, Wei Hu, Yong Long, Franklin R. Tay, and Jihua Chen. "Associations Among Bruxism, Gastroesophageal Reflux Disease, and Tooth Wear." *Journal of Clinical Medicine* 7, no. 11 (November 6, 2018): 417.

Klackenberg G. "Rhythmic Movements in Infancy and Early Childhood." *Acta Paediatrica Scand* 60, no. s224 (December 1971): 74–83.

Yeh, Shih-Bin, and Carlos H. Schenck. "Atypical Headbanging Presentation of Idiopathic Sleep Related Rhythmic Movement Disorder: Three Cases with Video-Polysomnographic Documentation." *Journal of Clinical Sleep Medicine* 8, no. 4 (August 2012): 403–11.

Vetrugno, Roberto, and Pasquale Montagna. "Sleep-to-Wake Transition Movement Disorders." *Sleep Medicine* 12, no. s2 (December 2011): S11–16.

DeCatanzaro, Denys A., and Graham Baldwin. "Effective Treatment of Self-Injurious Behavior through a Forced Arm Exercise." *American Journal of Mental Deficiency* 82, no. 5 (March 1978): 433–39.

Chapter 11: Restless Legs Syndrome/Periodic Limb Movement Disorder: *"If You Can't Sit Still During My Class, You Can Fidget Out in the Hall."*

Stubbs, Pamela Hamilton, and Arthur S. Walters. "Tools for the Assessment of Pediatric Restless Legs Syndrome." *Frontiers in Psychiatry* 11 (May 5, 2020): 356.

Pennestri, Marie-Hélène, Dominique Petit, Jean Paquet, Alex Desautels, Evelyne Touchette, Sylvana Côté, Richard E. Tremblay, Michel Boivin, and Jacques Montplaisir. "Childhood Restless Legs Syndrome: A Longitudinal Study of Prevalence and Familial Aggregation." *Journal of Sleep Research* (August 11, 2020): e13161.

American Academy of Sleep Medicine. *International classification of sleep disorders,* 3rd ed. Darien, USA. 2014.

Picchietti, Daniel L., Oliviero Bruni, Al de Weerd, Jeffrey S. Durmer, Suresh Kotagal, Judith A. Owens, and Narong Simakajornboon; International Restless Legs Syndrome Study Group (IRLSSG). "Pediatric Restless Legs Syndrome Diagnostic Criteria: An Update by the International Restless Legs Syndrome Study Group." *Sleep Medicine* 14, no. 12 (December 2013): 1253–59.

Ahmed, Nada, Mohamed Kandil, Mohamed Elfil, Abdalla Jamal, and Brian B. Koo. "Hypothyroidism in Restless Legs Syndrome." *Journal of Sleep Research* (June 1, 2020): e13091.

Trenkwalder, Claudia, Richard Allen, Birgit Högl, Walter Paulus, and Juliane Winkelmann. "Restless Legs Syndrome Associated with Major Diseases: A Systematic Review and New Concept." *Neurology* 86, no. 14 (April 5, 2016): 1336–43.

DelRosso, Lourdes M., and Raffaele Ferri. "The Prevalence of Restless Sleep Disorder Among a Clinical Sample of Children and Adolescents Referred to a Sleep Centre." *Journal of Sleep Research* 28, no. 6 (December 2019): e12870.

DelRosso, Lourdes M., Raffaele Ferri, Richard P. Allen, Oliviero Bruni, Diego Garcia-Borreguero, Suresh Kotagal, Judith A. Owens, Patricio Peirano, Narong Simakajornboon, and Daniel L. Picchietti; International Restless Legs Syndrome Study Group (IRLSSG). "Consensus Diagnostic Criteria for a Newly Defined Pediatric Sleep Disorder: Restless Sleep Disorder (RSD)." *Sleep Medicine* 75 (November 2020): 335–40.

Chapter 12: Enuresis: *Despite What Your Pediatrician Keeps Telling You, This Is Not Normal!*

Sá, Cacilda Andrade, Ana Carolina Gusmão Paiva, Maria Clotilde Lima Bezerra de Menezes, Liliana Fajardo de Oliveira, Carlos Augusto Gomes, André Avarese de Figueiredo, José de Bessa, and José Murillo B. Netto. "Increased Risk of Physical Punishment Among Enuretic Children with Family History of Enuresis." *Journal of Urology* 195, no. 4, pt. 2 (April 2016): 1227–30.

Richardson, Anne Steese. *Better Babies and Their Care.* New York: Frederick A. Stokes, 1914.

Wan, Julian, and Saul Greenfield. "Enuresis and Common Voiding Abnormalities." *Pediatric Clinics of North America* 44, no. 5 (October 1997): 1117–31.

Yousef, Khalida Anwer, Huda O. Basaleem, and Mariam Taher bin Yahiya. "Epidemiology of Nocturnal Enuresis in Basic Schoolchildren in Aden Governorate, Yemen." *Saudi Journal of Kidney Diseases and Transplantation* 22, no. 1 (January 2011): 167–73.

Nevéus, Tryggve. "Pathogenesis of Enuresis: Towards a New Understanding." *International Journal of Urology* 23, no. 3 (March 2017): 174–82.

Ferrara, Pietro, Roberta Autuori, Flavia Dosa, Alessandro Di Lucia, Antonio Gatto, and Antonio Chiaretti. "Medical Comorbidity of Nocturnal Enuresis in Children." *Indian Journal of Nephrology* 29, no. 5 (September–October 2019): 345–52.

Esmael, Ahmed, Mohammed Elsherief, Mohamed Abdelsalam, Lotfy Bendary, and Hossam Egila. "Sleep Architecture in Valproate-Induced Nocturnal Enuresis in Primary School and Preschool Children." *Journal of Child Neurology* 35, no. 14 (December 2020): 975–82.

Wolfish, Norman M., R. Terry Pivik, and Keith A. Busby. "Elevated Sleep Arousal Thresholds in Enuretic Boys: Clinical Implications." *Acta Paediatrica* 86, no. 4 (April 1997): 381–84.

Dhondt, Karlien, Ann Raes, Piet Hoebeke, Erik Van Laecke, Charlotte Van Herzeele, and Johan Vande Walle. "Abnormal Sleep Architecture and Refractory Nocturnal Enuresis." *Journal of Urology* 182, no. S4 (October 2009): 1961–65.

Monda, Jeffrey M., and Douglas A. Husmann. "Primary Nocturnal Enuresis: A Comparison Among Observation, Imipramine, Desmopressin Acetate and Bed-Wetting Alarm Systems." *Journal of Urology* 154, no. 2, pt. 2 (August 1995): 745–48.

Ravanshad, Yalda, Anoush Azarfar, Mohammad Esmaeeli, Zahra Mostafavian, Elham Zahabi, and Sahar Ravanshad. "Effect of Low Dose Imipramine in Patients with Nocturnal Enuresis, a Randomized Clinical Trial." *Iran Journal of Kidney Diseases* 13, no. 4 (July 2019): 257–61.

Jalkut, Mark W., Steven E. Lerman, and Bernard M. Churchill. "Enuresis." *Pediatric Clinics of North America* 48, no. 6 (December 2001): 1461–88.

Edwards, S. D , and H. I. van der Spuy. "Hypnotherapy as a Treatment for Enuresis." *Journal of Child Psychology and Psychiatry* 26, no. 1 (January 1985): 161–70.

Jeyakumar, Anita, Syed I. Rahman, Eric S. Armbrecht, and Ron Mitchell. "The Association between Sleep-Disordered Breathing and Enuresis in Children." *Laryngoscope* 122, no. 8 (August 2012): 1873–77.

Dhondt, Karlien, Elien Baert, Charlotte Van Herzeele, Ann Raes, Luitzen-Albert Groen, Piet Hoebeke, and Johan Vande Walle. "Sleep Fragmentation and Increased Periodic Limb Movements Are More Common in Children with Nocturnal Enuresis." *Acta Paediatrica* 103, no. 6 (June 2014): e268–72.

Kinsey, Alfred C., Wardell B. Pomeroy, and Clyde E. Martin. *Sexual Behavior in the Human Male*. Philadelphia: W. B. Saunders, 1948.

Chapter 13: Snoring and Sleep Apnea: *"He Has Grandma's Eyes and Grandpa's Compromised Breathing."*

Brietzke, Scott E., Eliot S. Katz, and David W. Roberson. "Can History and Physical Examination Reliably Diagnose Pediatric Obstructive Sleep Apnea/Hypopnea

Syndrome? A Systematic Review of the Literature." *Otolaryngology—Head and Neck Surgery* 131, no. 6 (December 2004): 827–32.

Zancanella, Edilson, F. M. Haddad, L. A. Oliveira, A. Nakasato, Bruno Bernardo Duarte, Carolina Ferraz de Paula Soares, Michel Burihan Cahali, Alan Luiz Eckeli, Bruno Caramelli, L. F. Drager, B. D. Ramos, M. Nóbrega, Simone C. Fagondes, and Nathalia C. Andrada; Associação Brasileira de Otorrinolaringologia e Cirurgia Cérvico-Facial; Academia Brasileira de Neurologia; Sociedade Brasileira de Cardiologia; Sociedade Brasileira de Pediatria; Sociedade Brasileira de Pneumologia e Tisiologia. "Obstructive Sleep Apnea and Primary Snoring: Diagnosis." *Brazilian Journal of Otorhinolaryngology* 80, no. S1 (January–February 2014): S1–16.

Chapter 14: Sleep and Special Situations:
You Are Now Entering a World of Total Medical Confusion and Misinformation. Please Buckle Up.

Simpson, Ryne, Anthony A. Oyekan, Zarmina Ehsan, and David G. Ingram. "Obstructive Sleep Apnea in Patients with Down Syndrome: Current Perspectives." *Nature and Science of Sleep* 10 (September 13, 2018): 287–93.

Reynolds, Ann M., Gnakub N. Soke, Katherine R. Sabourin, Susan Hepburn, Terry Katz, Lisa D. Wiggins, Laura A. Schieve, and Susan E. Levy. "Sleep Problems in 2- to 5-Year-Olds with Autism Spectrum Disorder and Other Developmental Delays." *Pediatrics* 143, no. 3 (March 2019): e20180492.

Malow, Beth A., Mary L. Marzec, Susan G. McGrew, Lily Wang, Lynette M. Henderson, and Wendy L. Stone. "Characterizing Sleep in Children with Autism Spectrum Disorders: A Multidimensional Approach." *Sleep* 29, no. 12 (December 2006): 1563–71.

Souders, Margaret C., Thorton B. A. Mason, Otto Valladares, Maja Bucan, Susan E. Levy, David S. Mandell, Terri E. Weaver, and Jennifer Pinto-Martin. "Sleep Behaviors and Sleep Quality in Children with Autism Spectrum Disorders." *Sleep* 32, no. 12 (December 2009): 1566–78.

Mazurek, Micah O., and Kristin Sohl. "Sleep and Behavioral Problems in Children with Autism Spectrum Disorder." *Journal of Autism and Developmental Disorders* 46, no. 6 (June 2016): 1906–15.

Kanney, Michelle L., Jeffrey S. Durmer, Lynn Marie Trotti, and Roberta Leu. "Rethinking Bedtime Resistance in Children with Autism: Is Restless Legs Syndrome to Blame?" *Journal of Clinical Sleep Medicine* 16, no. 12 (December 2020): 2029–35.

Shamsaei, Farshid, Samira Yadollahifar, and Amir Sadeghi. "Relationship Between Sleep Quality and Quality of Life in Patients with Bipolar Disorder." *Sleep Science* 13, no. 1 (2020): 65–69.

Stanislaus, Sharleny, Maj Vinberg, Sigurd Melbye, Mads Frost, Jonas Busk, Jakob E. Bardram, Lars Vedel Kessing, and Maria Faurholt-Jepsen. "Smartphone-Based Activity Measurements in Patients with Newly Diagnosed Bipolar Disorder, Unaffected Relatives and Control Individuals." *International Journal of Bipolar Disorders* 8, no. 1 (November 2, 2020): 32.

Zangani, Caroline, Cecilia Casetta, Alejandro Serrano Saunders, Francesco Donati, Eleonora Maggioni, and Armando D'Agostino. "Sleep Abnormalities Across Different Clinical Stages of Bipolar Disorder: A Review of EEG Studies." *Neuroscience & Biobehavioral Reviews* 118 (November 2020): 247–57.

Montgomery, Paul, Jennifer R. Burton, Richard P. Sewell, Thees F. Spreckelsen, and Alexandra J. Richardson. "Fatty Acids and Sleep in UK Children: Subjective and Pilot Objective Sleep Results from the DOLAB Study—A Randomized Controlled Trial." *Journal of Sleep Research* 23, no. 4 (August 2014): 364–88.

Chapter 15: Disorders of Fatigue:
Why Your Kid Is Exhausted (and Not Depressed)

Jason, Leonard A., Meredyth Evans, Molly Brown, and Nicole Porter. "What Is Fatigue? Pathological and Nonpathological Fatigue." *PM&R* 2, no. 5 (May 2010): 327–31.

Centers for Disease Control and Prevention. "What Is ME/CFS?" Atlanta: Centers for Disease Control and Prevention, US Department of Health and Human Services; 2020, accessed April 29, 2021, https://www.cdc.gov/me-cfs/about /index.html.

Yancey, Joseph R., and Sarah M. Thomas. "Chronic Fatigue Syndrome: Diagnosis and Treatment." *American Family Physician* 86, no. 8 (October 15, 2012): 741–46.

Chapter 16: Time to See a Sleep Specialist:
Pediatric Sleep Doctor—It's Totally a Real Thing!

Kang, Peter B., James F. Bale Jr., Mark Mintz, Sucheta M. Joshi, Donald L. Gilbert, Carrie Radabaugh, Holly Ruch-Ross, Section on Neurology Executive Committee of the American Academy of Pediatrics, and the Board of Directors of the Child Neurology Society. "The Child Neurology Clinical Workforce in 2015: Report of the AAP/CNS Joint Taskforce." *Neurology* 87, no. 13 (September 27, 2016): 1384–92.

Appendix B

Turner D. "A Review of the Use of Modafinil for Attention-Deficit Hyperactivity Disorder." *Expert Rev Neurother* 6, no. 4 (April 2006): 455–68.

Index

About the Author

Chris Winter is a sleep specialist and neurologist who has been involved in sleep research and the practice of sleep medicine in one way or another since 1992. He sees kids and adults in his sleep clinic, works to help professional sports teams sleep better, and is the author of the book *The Sleep Solution: Why Your Sleep Is Broken and How to Fix It*. He resides in Charlottesville, Virginia, with his wife and kids and loves to travel when he can get them all together.